Lecture Notes
in Business Information Processing

409

Series Editors

Wil van der Aalst
RWTH Aachen University, Aachen, Germany
John Mylopoulos
University of Trento, Trento, Italy
Michael Rosemann
Queensland University of Technology, Brisbane, QLD, Australia
Michael J. Shaw
University of Illinois, Urbana-Champaign, IL, USA
Clemens Szyperski
Microsoft Research, Redmond, WA, USA

More information about this series at http://www.springer.com/series/7911

Steven Mertens

Enabling Process Management for Loosely Framed Knowledge-intensive Processes

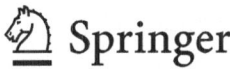 Springer

Steven Mertens ⓘ
Ghent University
Ghent, Belgium

ISSN 1865-1348   ISSN 1865-1356   (electronic)
Lecture Notes in Business Information Processing
ISBN 978-3-030-66192-2   ISBN 978-3-030-66193-9   (eBook)
https://doi.org/10.1007/978-3-030-66193-9

Preface

"A PhD is like childbirth for the brain"
"How hard can it be? Mind-meltingly, stomach-churningly, sleep-deprivingly difficult"
Emma Jane, The Punch/PerthNow (2011)

If you don't have a PhD: yes, this statement is accurate. A little sympathy wouldn't hurt, you know.

If you're currently doing a PhD: your brain is probably already pregnant. I feel you. Every day it gets a little harder to drag your ailing body out of bed. Dealing with the occasional morning sickness (unrelated to last night's drinking). The prospect of the dreaded third trimester looming (i.e., writing the book and numerous postdoc proposals). Maybe it's not too late to consider a late-term abortion?

If you have a PhD: congratulations! You won... Erm... Well what did you win? I guess you can proudly call yourself a doctor. However, don't bother getting up when someone yells out for a doctor on a plane. They will not be as impressed with the highest academic degree as one might expect.

Now skip past the rest of this preface section, read this book from cover to cover, and only afterwards return here to read the rest. No cheating! You will be quizzed!

Who am I kidding? You're probably not actually going to bother with the rest of this book. Just like if I would be presenting you my newborn, you're going to congratulate me and disappear as soon as you get a whiff of its insides...

How about trying to imagine reading this book from cover to cover? It's over 200 pages of scientific and peer-reviewed work. That's a lot, right? Now imaging having to write such a behemoth. Each chapter/paper needs a problem statement, relevant research questions, a methodology to find answers to those questions, a literature review of the state-of-the-art on the subject and, most importantly, a description of actual contributions to that state-of-the-art. Each chapter/section/paragraph/sentence/word carefully written, criticized by peers, rewritten, criticized by peers, rewritten again, criticized by peers, etc. until everyone involved starts to involuntarily cringe at the mere thought of it. But you can't just start writing. A paper is merely a report of research that you would've already done by then. The research consists of formulating interesting, relevant, and unsolved problems, which you subsequently must tackle head-on – fully aware of the fact that it had probably already crossed the minds of other researchers, who had likely discarded the idea because they considered it an insurmountable problem that only fools would waste their time on. And yet again, you cannot just start formulating interesting, relevant, and unsolved problems without being an expert on a certain subject. How do you become an expert? Reading, more reading, even more reading and – you've guessed it – some more reading (my favorite pastime!). Luckily, you can stop when you've learned enough buzzwords to fool other researchers into thinking that you know what you're talking about. Fake it till you make it! After all, we're living in the Trump-era...

"I know words, I have the best words"
Donald J. Trump, 45th president of the United States of America

But before you can start reading up on a certain subject, you need to choose a suitable subject. Something that interests you in a domain with unresolved problems. Problems that are not only practically relevant – your own prerequisite – but also academically relevant. And most importantly, problems for which your particular set of skills could actually be an asset.

"...what I do have are a very particular set of skills; skills I have acquired over a very long [academic] career. Skills that make me a nightmare for people like you [the audience]."
Bryan Mills (played by Liam Neeson) – Taken (2008)

This requires long days of introspective thinking – trying to come up with something that no one else has already done or is currently working on. And then, a eureka-moment! A surefire Nobel prize winning idea! As soon as possible, you meet with your promotors to blow their mind with your amazing idea, only to be met with a lot less enthusiasm than you were expecting. Instead they point out all the (obvious) holes in your idea, while trying to maintain a constructive façade as to not discourage you too much. And this is repeated several times until you find yourself on the couch. Watching House M.D. on TV. Tired of the search. Writing a report on genetic programming for a mandatory course. Thinking that a PhD might not be in your wheelhouse. And then suddenly it hits you. You like watching House M.D., Dr. Gregory House and his team work in a chaotic manner (lacking any type of process support), your research group covers process management and you're currently writing a report on a technique that can search through a chaotic mess and find good solutions. And so, the seed for this dissertation was planted. It germinated. Its roots took hold. A seedling saw the light. A mighty tree grew. And then they cut it down to print this book.

If you're still reading this: thank you for already making it this far. Mind you, you're still 11 pages removed from the actual first page, but don't let that discourage you. Maybe it will be all worth it. At least I can say that it was worth it for me. The last 6 years have been great, albeit with some unavoidable ups and downs. I got to keep calling myself a student, and sometimes act like one (anyone up for a midweek night out?), even though my bank account kept getting a nice monthly refill. I got to travel and see some beautiful places. And, of course, work with and around some amazing people. First off, I would like to thank my promotors Frederik and Geert for their unwavering support and for creating a great working environment. My jury members Amy, Diederik, Fernanda, Niels, and Melissa for all their valuable input and questions. An extra thank you to Melissa for using her connections to get us started in the healthcare domain, and to Diederik for his willingness to hear us out, to try to understand our ambitious and overly technical ideas from the get-go, and for providing us with opportunities that would have never been possible otherwise. And then all my other colleagues... Words cannot express my gratitude and the utter pleasure it was spending the last few years with you all, so no point in trying (right?): Aygun,

Bambang, Ben, David, Dirk, Dries, Georgios, Gert, Griet, Jan, Jana, Laleh, Machteld, Maria, Martine, Miao, Michael, Miljace, Mohanad, Nadia, Pooyan, Renata, Sven, Tahir, Thiago and Camilla, Thomas, Tom, Xiaji, and everyone from the second floor (too many to name). And finally, I would like to thank my family and friends for putting up with me, for their continuous support, and for providing me with a timely distraction when it was needed the most.

"Perhaps childbirth is not that bad after all – some people just like to exaggerate."
Steven Mertens (childless and full of male ignorance) – October 2019

Contents

Chapter 1
Introduction

1.1 Introduction

1.1.1 Terminology and Research Context

This PhD addresses shortcomings that relate to the process orientation and support in settings that house loosely framed knowledge-intensive processes. Before diving into the problem, we will first briefly describe the general domain, the characteristics of the target processes and the architecture of the tool support.

Business Process Management (BPM) is the field that researches how consistent outcomes can be achieved and continuously improved by managing the way work is performed in an organization [1, 2]. The way of performing work is captured in the concept of a **business process**, which is a collection of inter-related events, activities, decision points and actors that collectively deliver value to customers or realize a business goal [3–5]. Therefore, BPM is defined as a body of concepts, methods, techniques and tools to support the design, configuration, discovery, analysis, redesign, execution and monitoring of business processes [1].

A possible way of classifying business processes is according to their predictability[1] [6, 7]. First, a **tightly framed** process is always executed in just one of a few predefined, consistent and unambiguous ways (e.g., the mass production of electronics). When the process is less structured it is called **loosely framed or flexible**, which entails that a process is executed in a large, but finite and predefined, number of ways (e.g., the treatment of patients in a hospital). Next, a process is **ad hoc framed** if it is typically executed starting from a predefined process model, but ad hoc changes occur frequently during the execution. This leads to the models being used only once or perhaps a few times before being discarded or changed (e.g., project planning). Lastly, **unframed** processes are processes where each execution is unique and generally impossible to predefine (e.g., groupware systems).

---

[1]Predictability of the actual processes, not of models made of the processes!

© Springer Nature Switzerland AG 2020
S. Mertens: Enabling Process Management for Loosely Framed
Knowledge-Intensive Processes, LNBIP 409,
https://doi.org/10.1007/978-3-030-66193-9_1

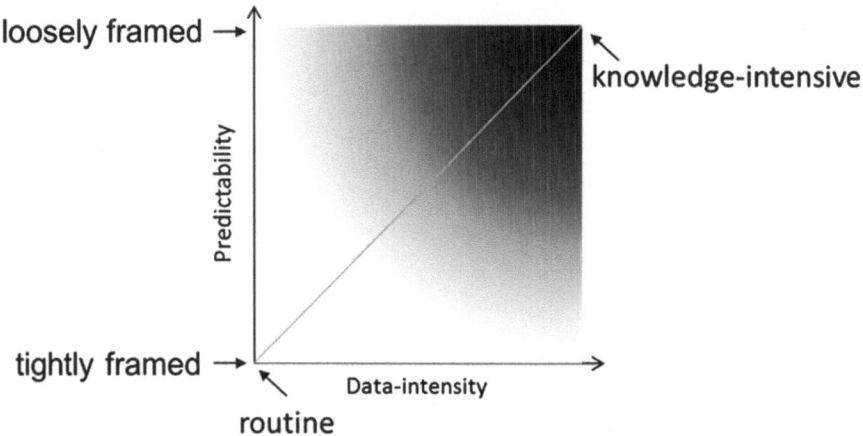

Fig. 1.1 Classification of processes according to the predictability and the data-intensity

This classification according to the predictability of processes can be further complemented with a data-intensity dimension (see Fig. 1.1). The data is linked to the choice for a certain the process variation, and therefore, becomes more and more relevant as the predictability decreases. The scale ranging from tightly framed to unframed processes typically corresponds to processes becoming more and more data-intensive (gray diagonal in Fig. 1.1) [7]. Processes situated in the lower left corner of Fig. 1.1 have few variations and no or some simple decisions (e.g., manufacturing processes), while processes in the upper right corner have many variations and many complex decisions (e.g., the diagnosis and treatment of patients in a hospital). Off-diagonal processes are certainly possible, but rather the exception than the rule. Processes situated in the lower right corner have few variations but complex decisions (e.g., the loan approval process in a bank), while processes in the upper left corner have many variations but no or just a few simple decisions (e.g., a 'naïve' theme park experience, where all rides are an option all the time).

The dark area in Fig. 1.1 corresponds to what are defined as **Knowledge-intensive Processes** (KiPs). These are business processes whose conduct and execution are heavily dependent on knowledge workers performing various interconnected knowledge-intensive decision-making tasks [6, 8]. KiPs are genuinely knowledge-, information- and data-intensive and require substantial flexibility at design- and run-time. Many ad hoc framed and unframed processes can also be regarded as KiPs but are out of scope of this dissertation, because the lack of framing (i.e., cannot predefine the activities and process variations) means that they require a different management approach.

The application of BPM in organizations can be mapped to the phases of the **BPM lifecycle** (see Fig. 1.2), which encompasses a range of methods and tools to identify processes and to manage individual processes [1]. It starts with the **identification** of the processes related to a specific business problem. In the next phase, process **discovery**, the current state of the relevant identified processes is documented in

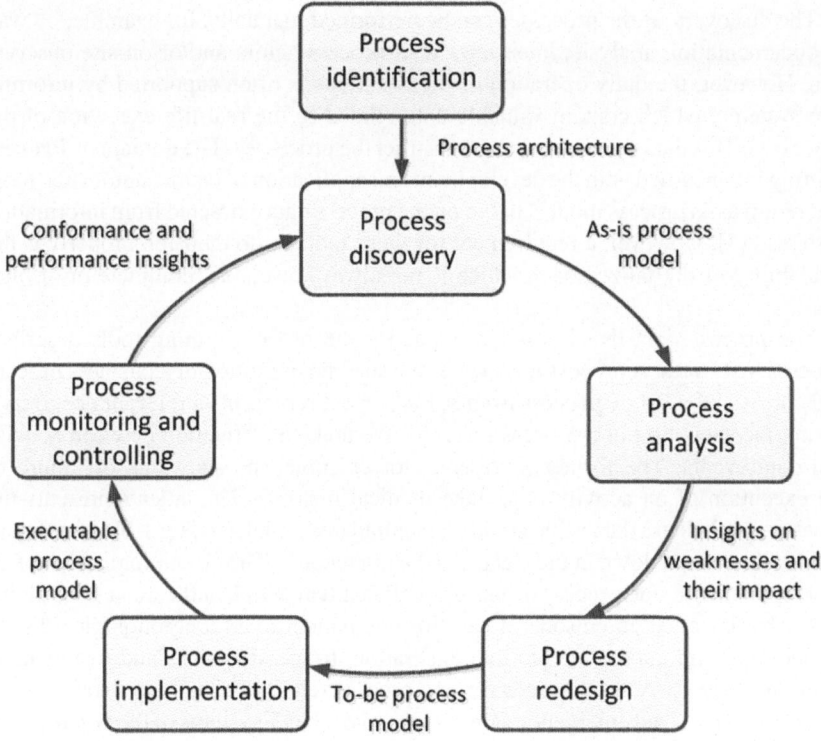

Fig. 1.2 The BPM lifecycle (Fig. 1.7 from [1])

the form of (as-is) models. Issues in the current state will subsequently be identified, documented and quantified as part of the process **analysis** phase. In the phase that follows, changes to counter the issues are identified and compared. The most promising change options are combined to **redesign** the processes. The proposed changes will then need to be **implemented** in the form of organizational changes and/or process automation. Once the redesigned processes are up and running, relevant data will be collected and analyzed to evaluate the impact of the changes on the identified process issues during the **monitoring and controlling** phase. And it does not end here. New issues may arise in the redesigned or other processes of the organization. Therefore, the BPM lifecycle is a cycle that needs to be repeated on a continuous basis.

Starting from the process discovery phase onwards, a representation is needed of the identified processes. **Business Process Modeling** entails the explicit representation of business processes by describing its activities, events/states, and control-flow logic [9]. Such representation is called a process model. These models can subsequently be used as a way of documenting a process, as a way of representing the as-is and to-be situations, as a means to check conformance and/or as a precise schedule for the execution of the process [10].

The discovery of the processes can be performed manually, for example, by way of documentation analysis, interviews with process actors and/or on-site observation. However, the daily operation of organizations is often supported by information systems, which contain valuable data related to the real-life execution of the processes. This data can be used to reconstruct the processes. The domain of **Process Mining** is concerned with the development and application of (semi-)automated tools that return as-is process models based on the process data extracted from information systems [11]. However, a requirement for these tools to do their job properly is the availability of digitalized data, which is not always available, complete or of high quality.

The process data that is used as input for the process mining tools describes **process instances**. A process instance is one specific execution of a business process and consists of a list of **process events**. Each event represents a relevant occurrence during the execution of a process instance. We make a distinction between activity and data events. The former represents, for example, the start, end or failure of the execution of an activity (e.g., take medical history). The latter represents the timestamp of when a data value is added, manipulated or deleted (e.g., 'blood pressure of 140/90' written down in the electronic health record). The chronological list of all events relating to one process instance is called a **trace**. In healthcare, a trace aligns with what is called an episode of care for one patient (e.g., a chronological list of all activities and data related to the registration, triage, diagnosis and treatment of a certain patient). A set of traces for one process (e.g., a collection of traces of all patients that received emergency care) as logged by the IT systems of the organization is called an **event log**. To make such an event log, data first needs to be extracted and combined from the data sources that span the information system of the organization. The resulting data should subsequently be filtered and preprocessed into an event stream format.

The process implementation phase of the BPM lifecycle covers two aspects: organizational change management and process automation [1]. In this dissertation, the focus will be on the side of process automation. More specifically, process automation supported by the use of a **Business Process Management System** (BPMS) (a.k.a. Process Aware Information System). A BPMS is a generic software system that coordinates the enactment of business processes involving people, applications and/or information sources based on process models [3, 12]. This definition was later expanded to define the BPMS as a more general collection of components that serve the goal of managing business processes (traditional BPMS in Fig. 1.3) [13]. The components of a BPMS are:

- The **Business Process Design**-component allows users to view, create and modify the business process models used by the BPMS. This component relates to the process discovery and redesign phases of the BPM lifecycle.
- The **Business Process Engine**-component (BPE): is responsible for the correct enactment of process models. This component relates to the process implementation and, to a lesser extent, the controlling and monitoring phases of the BPM lifecycle.

- The **Business Process Analytics**-component enables analysis of the process models, the executing/historic process instances and simulations. Typically, the results of these analyses are presented as a process dashboard or in reports. This component relates to the process analysis and the controlling and monitoring phases of the BPM lifecycle.
- The **Business Process Monitoring**-component monitors the execution of running process instances. This is often in terms of Key Performance Indicators (KPIs), but more advanced features such as predictions of potentially unwanted future behavior or outcomes are also possible. This component relates to the process controlling and monitoring phase of the BPM lifecycle.
- The **Business Process Exception Handling**-component is responsible for how the BPMS handles process exceptions (i.e., deviations from the given process models) in real-time. This component does not directly relate to any of the BPM lifecycle phases but can be regarded as a fail-safe to handle new or unidentified process issues. The invocation of this component should be the starting point for a new iteration of the lifecycle.
- The **Business Process Simulation**-component offers simulations based on a given process model and stochastic functions for the other parameters. It can be used to analyze the dynamic behavior of the process over time. This component relates to the process analysis and redesign phases of the BPM lifecycle.

Process discovery is often already being applied in the context of a traditional BPMS-components and serves the goal of managing business processes as was put forward as the idea behind the original expansion of the BPMS responsibilities. As a result, we will also include a **Business Process Discovery**-component, which supports methods for process (and decision) discovery from a given event log. The

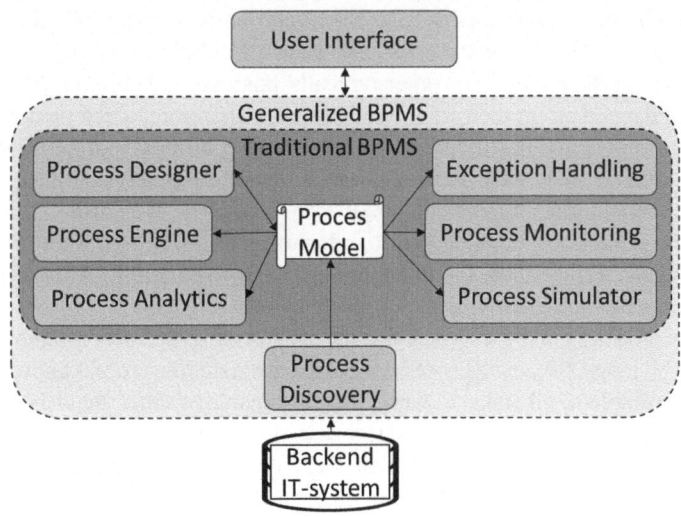

Fig. 1.3 The traditional and generalized architecture of a BPMS

resulting model can be used as input for the other components. Figure 1.3 presents the components of a traditional (extended) and of a generalized BPMS that includes this extra component.

1.1.2 Problem Statement

This dissertation started from an observed lack of a BPM framework for loosely framed KiPs. The characteristics of these processes have proven to be a formidable obstacle to the successful adoption of BPM to those settings [6]. On the one hand, their loosely framed nature leads to processes where deviations and variations are the norm rather than the exception. Therefore, most, if not all, of these process variations need to be accounted for one way or the other by the framework to be able to provide the necessary **flexibility**. On the other hand, their knowledge-intensive nature stems from the need to choose a process variation for each process instance. Each variation applies to a certain setting, and the process actors, also called knowledge workers, need to decide which one they find appropriate for the process instance at hand. The immense number of process variations means that the amount of knowledge needed to distinguish between them is also immense.

The knowledge of knowledge workers is often referred to as **tacit knowledge**, in that it primarily resides in some implicit form in their memory [6]. Loosely framed KiPs often also have a **dynamic** component [14]. The knowledge needed to execute the process as well as the acceptable process variations can evolve over time (e.g., medical procedures can change due to new insights or technological advancements). This further exacerbates the problem of knowledge remaining tacit, because efforts to document it are confronted with a heavy struggle to stay up to date. This also applies to the knowledge workers themselves. Not everyone is as aware of every novelty, which potentially leads to differences in how each would handle a certain situation. Additionally, each knowledge worker typically possesses a subset of the total tacit knowledge dependent on their role in the process. Therefore, a complete picture of the process knowledge is only possible by combining all pieces of knowledge, like pieces of a puzzle, without a guarantee that there will not be any conflicts. This also causes personnel turnover to be potentially very disruptive, even disastrous, because it is unclear what knowledge each of the departing knowledge workers possessed. That knowledge is inevitably lost and there is no way to determine whether potential replacements can sufficiently make up for this loss.

Process modeling provides a medium for transforming tacit process knowledge to explicit knowledge, because a process model encapsulates the process knowledge and makes it available to all stakeholders. This also enables further analysis to correct, redesign and optimize the process. However, the need for flexibility, the lack of transparency and the dynamic nature of these processes also hinder the adoption of process modeling techniques. In the medical sector, they have tried to sidestep these issues with the use of clinical pathways (CPs) and similar concepts like clinical guidelines, critical pathways, integrated care pathways and care maps. Although the exact definition of what they entail can vary from paper to paper [15], the general consensus seems to be that they are best practice schedules of medical and nursing procedures for the treatment of patients with a specific pathology (e.g., breast cancer). CPs can be considered process models, but real-life situations are typically much more complex. Comorbidities and practical limitations (e.g., resource availability) can prevent CPs from being implemented as-is. The real process also comprises more than just the treatment of patients because activities to try and reach a diagnosis and other practicalities should be considered as well. A CP is therefore a form of high-level model of one idealized process variation. Modeling every process variation explicitly is easy for tightly framed processes, where there are only a couple of variations possible. This referred to as **imperative modeling** (e.g., BPMN) and is used to explicitly specify all allowed behavior. However, the numerous acceptable process variations of loosely framed processes make this approach less suitable for loosely framed processes.

The lack of a suitable process modeling language also severely inhibits the development of any kind of **operational process support** for these processes. The BPE-component of a BPMS requires a process model to provide users with information and support on how they can proceed during the execution of a process. In the current situation, process support for loosely framed KiPs typically ranges from non-existent to rudimentary at most. A process model is almost never available to serve as a foundation to offer support or assistance. Therefore, knowledge workers are currently left to their own devices, but they are still expected to execute the process instances in a satisfactory manner. This puts a lot of responsibility and pressure on the knowledge workers. The result is a process that scores very bad when it comes to **transparency**. This lack of transparency is also a barrier to analysis and optimization, which in turn can lead to questions about the unmeasurable efficiency.

1.1.3 Research Objectives

The general objective of this dissertation is the development of a BPMS for loosely framed KiPs. It should support the different phases of the BPM lifecycle as described in Sect. 1.1. In the scope of this dissertation, we will focus on the development of the main components of such a system: the Process Designer-, Discovery-, Engine- and Analysis-components.

> **General objective: The development of a BPMS for loosely framed KiPs**

The Process Designer-component requires a process modeling language that suits loosely framed KiPs. **Declarative modeling languages** (e.g., Declare) take on the opposite viewpoint of imperative languages: the outside-in approach. They describe the rules and constraints by which the process variations must abide [16]. The unwanted process variations are prohibited based on these rules and constraints, while all other variations are allowed implicitly and without having to enumerate each valid variations [17].

Although the basic principles behind declarative process modeling languages are well suited to model loosely framed KiPs [7, 16, 18], the suitability of a specific declarative language also depends on the availability and expressive power of each of the necessary business process modeling perspectives [19]. First, the **functional** (i.e., the available activities/events and their instances) and **control-flow** (i.e., restrictions on when activities/events occur) perspectives are the core of a process modeling language. For declarative languages, these two perspectives provide an innate support for the 'flexibility by design'-principle [20] that is essential to model the flow of activities in loosely framed KiPs. Second, the 'knowledge' in KiPs alludes to the implicit or explicit knowledge needed by the process workers to execute the process. KiPs are governed by many rules and/or decisions processes [6, 21] and insight into these decisions is at least as important as what activities are available for execution. Modeling a decision process comes down to linking combinations of data values to some sort of outcome, which in turn requires a **data** perspective (a.k.a. information perspective). Third, resources play a vital role in loosely framed KiPs. Often, the execution of certain activities from the functional and control-flow perspectives depends on the availability of certain resources and those resources have certain properties expressed in data values (e.g., availability, speed, cost, quality, etc.) that influence the decisions in the data perspective of the process model. So, some form of **resource** perspective is also needed.

There exist several declarative process modeling languages, with the most popular being Declare [17, 22] and DCR Graphs [23]. The original definition of these languages addresses the functional and control-flow perspectives. Since then, several extensions have been proposed to increase the expressive power of these languages by adding additional functional and control-flow elements or adding new perspectives. However, none of the previously proposed declarative languages and extensions combines all the necessary perspectives for loosely framed KiPs.

> **Objective 1**: The development of a declarative process modeling language that suits loosely framed KiPs, which lays the foundation for the Process Designer-component of the BPMS

A suitable process modeling language for loosely framed KiPs creates an opportunity to gain insight into these processes. However, the difficulty now lies in finding the right approach to create the process models, as most of the process knowledge is of a tacit nature. Traditionally, this is done by way of interviews with process actors and other domain experts. This is straightforward when there is little knowledge to extract, but otherwise can quickly become a very difficult, effort-intensive, time-consuming and error-prone task for both the modeler and the process actors. The inclusion of a process mining technique in the Process Discovery-component can provide an appealing alternative. It can offer a direct reflection of how things are actually done (i.e., an as-is process model), instead of an idealized description from interviews. Traditional process mining techniques automatically detect control-flow patterns in a given dataset and turn these into a consistent process model that accurately reflects the process execution data.

Most process mining techniques assume an imperative viewpoint on the process. Recently, several declarative process mining techniques have been proposed [24–33]. The problem is that each of these techniques returns a process model written in one of the existing declarative process modeling languages or its extensions, and hence, not in the process modeling language that will be the result of objective 1. So, a new process mining technique is needed for the language definition of objective 1, which potentially could incorporate pieces of the existing declarative process mining techniques. In the context of loosely framed processes we are not just interested in mining the functional and control-flow perspectives, but also in a data perspective that contains the decision logic that governs the functional and control-flow perspectives. The automatically mining of a resource perspective is of lesser importance, because most organizational IT-systems do not log the data required (e.g., availabilities, authorization and usage), and will be regarded as future research.

The application of a process mining technique, which assumes that a satisfactory event log is available, is just one part of a larger method(ology) for process discovery. This method(ology) consists of the necessary steps to gather data, organize and process this data, the preparation of an event log that is aligned with the input requirements of the chosen process mining technique, the application of the process mining technique, a subsequent evaluation of the discovered model and iterative repetitions needed to obtain a satisfactory model. Two such methodologies have been proposed for imperative process discovery projects [34, 35], which focus on the functional and control-flow perspectives. However, a method for declarative process and decision discovery is still missing.

> <u>Objective 2</u>: The development of a method for process and decision discovery of loosely framed KiPs for the Process Discovery-component of the BPMS, and a corresponding mining technique that can mine a process and decision model from an event log

An accurate process model enables a deeper level of management and analysis. The question becomes how to use and leverage the model for the benefit of the process stakeholders. Declarative process modeling languages are known to be hard to understand by human actors [36]. The innate complexity of loosely framed KiPs only exacerbates this further. So, there is no point in putting a printed version of the process model, perhaps already redesigned or optimized, in the hands of the process actors and expecting them to enact it. However, computers are not bothered as much by this complexity, as long as the modeling language allows for an unambiguous interpretation of the models. They are much better at processing this type of information and certainly in these quantities. This is where the operational components of the BPMS come into play. The foundational architecture for traditional BPMS, called a workflow management system, was published in 1995 [37]. A process model serves as the input for such system and its components enable monitoring, management, analysis, optimization and simulation. Traditional BPMSs expect an imperative process model as input. These models have clearly defined paths that can be followed, whereas declarative process models just provide the rules for such valid paths but lack any sort of explicit definition. This difference has a profound impact on the requirements of some of the components of a BPMS.

For example, a traditional BPE simply must follow the explicitly defined paths of the given imperative model to determine the next and future activities. In contrast, a declarative process model does not define any explicit paths. The requirements for a BPE that executes declarative process models are therefore different and more complex, compared to a traditional BPE. A declarative BPE will first have to calculate which parts of the model apply to the context at hand. This filtered model subsequently enables the calculation of the activities that can be executed next, the activities that must eventually be executed and those that are prohibited either at specific moments or during the remainder of the process instance. It is of paramount importance that every path allowed/prohibited by the declarative process model is also allowed/prohibited by the BPE, to preserve the freedom to operate of the knowledge workers and prevent divergence from the model. When done correctly, this can significantly reduce the size of the set of rules that process actors get exposed to at one time, and thus, minimize the impact of the human understandability issues associated to declarative process models. The rules of the model that led to an activity being placed into one of the aforementioned categories can be made available to the process actors on-demand, exposing them to merely those pieces of the model that they require to accurately interpret it.

The intended BPE should be able to automatically interpret a given declarative process model, which relieves the process actors of this difficult and time-consuming task but offers little guidance when presented with the choice of multiple valid process variations. One way of offering guidance is to provide the process actor with analytical information on the available variations that can be used to rank them. This functionality is arguably not a part of the BPE-component itself, but rather of the Process Analytics-component of a BPMS as an additional layer on top of the BPE. The combination of these two subcomponents should provide rich operational support to process actors during the execution of a process instance. The BPE-component ensures that the execution conforms with the explicit knowledge of the given process and decision model, while the Process Analytics-component is used to offer insight and guidance.

> Objective 3: The development of a BPE- and Process Analytics-component for the BPMS that can offer support and guidance to process actors during the process execution

In summary, this dissertation will focus on the development of the core functionality of a generalized BPMS for loosely framed KiPs: the Process Designer-, Discovery-, Engine- and Analytics-components.

1.1.4 Research Methodology

The **Design Science Research** (DSR) methodology [38, 39] was applied in this research project, with an **Action Design Research** (ADR) cycle mixed in. DSR can be used to create and evaluate design artifacts such as constructs, models, methods and instantiations with scientific rigor [38]. Each artifact should solve one or more problems relevant to practice while the development and evaluation process should contribute new knowledge to the state of the art. DSR is inherently iterative and the creation of one artifact often requires the creation of nested artifacts. Therefore, it is best visualized using nested design cycles [40]. We make a distinction between two types of cycles: engineering and research cycles [41]. An engineering cycle (EC) consists of the necessary steps to design and evaluate an artefact to solve a well-defined problem. A research cycle (RC) is responsible for resolving a research related issue such as establishing the state of the art for a problem, finding and adapting related techniques, etc. Figure 1.4 presents an overview of the design cycles of this dissertation.

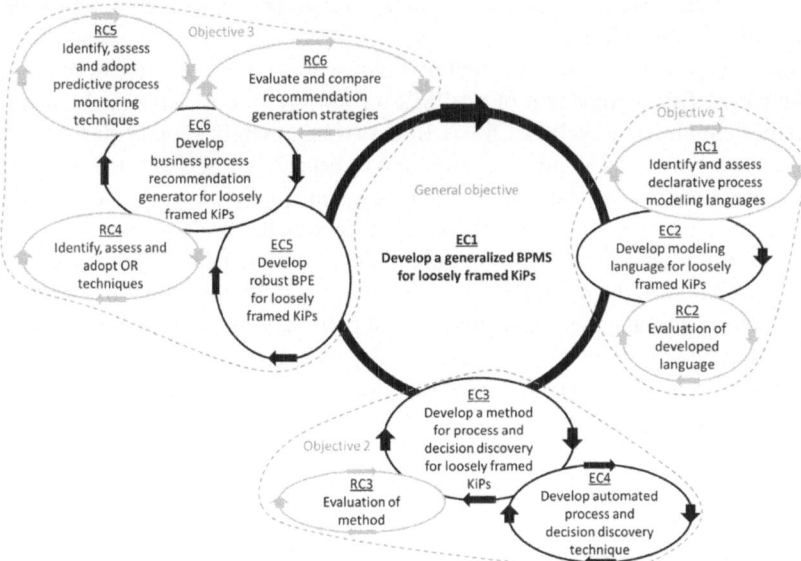

Fig. 1.4 The design science cycles of this dissertation and their relation to the research objectives (green dotted lines) (Color figure online)

The general objective from the previous section was translated to the main engineering cycle (EC1), which is responsible for developing a BPMS for loosely framed KiPs. This cycle had three smaller engineering cycles (EC2, EC3 and EC5).

EC2 was the translation of research objective 1, the development of a process modeling language for loosely framed KiPs and contained two smaller research cycles (RC1 and RC2). Literature already established that a modeling language that takes on a declarative viewpoint is preferable to one that takes on an imperative viewpoint. Therefore, RC1 was concerned with the identification and assessment of the existing declarative process modeling languages. The aspects of these languages that were deemed useful in the context of loosely framed KiPs were subsequently combined and extended in the continuation of EC2. The resulting process modeling language, called DeciClare, was then evaluated in RC2.

EC3 was the translation of research objective 2, the development of a method for process and decision discovery for loosely framed KiPs with a model written in the language developed in EC2 as output, and contained an engineering cycle (EC4) and a research cycle (RC3). We chose to apply ADR as methodology for EC3, which is a specific type of design science research for the design of research artifacts that explicitly provide theoretical contributions to the academic knowledge base, while simultaneously solving a practical problem [42]. Creating a process and decision model manually is unrealistic in practical settings for this type of processes. Therefore, an automated process and decision mining technique was first developed in EC4, which was a normal design science engineering cycle to start the ADR-cycle. The ADR-cycle itself focused on the development of the general discovery method, while simultaneously evaluating the method and mining technique by applying them to a real-life setting (RC3).

EC5 was the translation of the first part of research objective 3, the development of the robust BPE-component of a BPMS for loosely framed KiPs, and contained a smaller engineering cycle (EC6). A BPE that can merely support the execution of a declarative model is not very supportive, because loosely framed KiPs typically have a number of activities that can be executed next at any time during the execution of a process instance. Therefore, EC6 was the translation of the second part of research objective 3, the development of a recommendation generator for the BPE, and contained three smaller research cycles (RC4-RC6). During RC4 and RC5 we identified and assessed strategies from the operations research and predictive process monitoring domains that could be used to generate next-activity recommendations. The strategies that were deemed applicable, were subsequently implemented, evaluated and compared in RC6.

1.1.5 Dissertation Structure

This dissertation follows the structure of a paper-based dissertation, consisting of six chapters.

Chapter 1: Introduction

This chapter introduces the domain of process management, the targeted processes, the problems to be addressed, the research objectives and the chosen approach to achieve these objectives.

Chapter 2: Towards a Decision-aware Declarative Process Modeling Language for Knowledge-intensive Processes

This chapter is the result of the second iteration of RC1 and EC2, and the first iteration of RC2. It describes the development of a process modeling language for loosely framed KiPs.

Chapter 3: Discovering Loosely Framed Knowledge-intensive Processes using DeciClareMiner

This chapter is the result of EC4. It describes the development of an automated process and decision discovery technique for loosely framed KiPs.

Chapter 4: Integrated Declarative Process and Decision Discovery of the Emergency Care Process

This chapter is the result of EC3. It describes the development of a method for creating a process and decision knowledge base for loosely framed KiPs. The ADR-cycle combines the development of this method with the application of the process and decision discovery technique on real data from the emergency medicine department of a hospital (RC3).

Chapter 5: Operational Support for Loosely Framed Knowledge-intensive Processes

This chapter consists of two related parts. The first part is the result of EC5 and describes the development of a data-aware BPE that supports the execution of a declarative process model. The second part is the result of the first iteration of EC6 and RC4-6 and describes the evaluation and comparison of forty strategies to generate next-activity recommendations. The combination of these two subcomponents produces a fully operational BPE, which ensures that the process is executed in conformance to a given process model while also providing recommendations that support process actors during the execution of a process instance.

Chapter 6: Conclusion and Future Research

This chapter concludes the dissertation, discusses the generalizability of the results to other domains, lists the research contributions and implications for researchers and practitioners, and outlines possible future research opportunities.

Chapter 2
Towards a Decision-Aware Declarative Process Modeling Language for Knowledge-Intensive Processes

2.1 Introduction

A business process is a "collection of inter-related events, activities and decisions points that involve a number of actors and objects, and that collectively lead to an outcome that is of value to at least one customer" [1]. Business process modeling (BPM) is the practice of creating models that represent business processes [1, 3]. These models can subsequently be used as a way of documenting a process, as a way of representing the as-is and to-be situations, as a means to check conformance and/or as a precise schedule for the execution of the process [1]. Business process modeling is being applied in a variety of industries (e.g., manufacturing, insurance, utilities, retail, telecommunications, finance, etc.). As a result of the diversity in uses and target domains, a multitude of process modeling languages exist [7, 16, 43, 44]. Gantt and flow charts were part of the first wave and have since given way to modern-day techniques like BPMN [45], UML activity diagrams [46] and Declare [17, 22].

A possible way of classifying business processes is according to their *predictability* [6, 7]. First, a *tightly framed* process is always executed in just one of a few predefined, consistent and unambiguous ways (e.g., the mass production of electronics). When the process is less structured it is called *loosely framed*, which entails that a process is executed in a large, but finite and predefined, number of ways (e.g., the treatment of patients in a hospital). Next, a process is *ad hoc framed* if it is typically executed starting from a predefined process model, but ad hoc changes occur frequently during the execution. This leads to the models being used only once or perhaps a few times before being discarded or changed (e.g., project planning). Lastly, *unframed* processes are processes where each execution is unique and generally impossible to predefine (e.g., groupware systems). The scale ranging from tightly framed processes to unframed processes corresponds to processes becoming more and more knowledge-intensive [7]. Although there exist strongly framed processes that can be considered knowledge-intensive (e.g., the loan approval process in a

© Springer Nature Switzerland AG 2020
S. Mertens: Enabling Process Management for Loosely Framed
Knowledge-Intensive Processes, LNBIP 409,
https://doi.org/10.1007/978-3-030-66193-9_2

bank), these are more the exception rather than the rule. Di Ciccio, Marrella, et al. [6] define *knowledge-intensive business processes (KiPs)*, in general, as follows:

> *"Processes whose conduct and execution are heavily dependent on knowledge workers performing various interconnected knowledge-intensive decision-making tasks. KiPs are genuinely knowledge-, information- and data-intensive and require substantial flexibility at design- and run-time."*

The former part of this definition references the complex nature of these processes and the unmistakable human factor in all of this. The execution of the process is completely dependent on *knowledge workers* (e.g., doctors), who each use their specific knowledge to contribute to the process. This knowledge is a form of processed information (i.e., understood patterns) and information (i.e., detected patterns) can be defined as data values (i.e., raw data) with a certain meaning or purpose [47]. So, in essence, modeling knowledge requires the modeling language to support at least a *data* perspective (i.e., the available data records, attributes, values and their relationships). The latter part of the definition references the loosely framed to unframed nature of most KiPs. A knowledge worker (i.e., part of the *resource* perspective with the available resources and their relationships) requires a significant amount of freedom to operate, so that he or she can apply their knowledge to specific contexts. This freedom can be incorporated at design-time, at run-time or both [8]. For example, a model can explicitly specify a decision point and a specific process variation for each decision outcome at design-time or even leave these underspecified to be determined at run-time. Basically, this part of the definition indicates that a *functional* (i.e., the available activities/events and their instances) and *control-flow* perspective (i.e., restrictions on when activities/events occur) are integral parts of a modeling language for KiPs to be able to cater to this need for flexibility.

The classification can now be translated to a classification based on the relative importance of the functional, control-flow, resource and data perspectives to the process. For tightly framed processes the focus is mainly on precise definition of the functional and control-flow perspectives, and in some cases also on the resource perspectives [6]. However, for loosely framed processes the data perspective is at least of equal importance as the other perspectives, because it is an essential requirement to model the knowledge that governs the other perspectives [6]. The other perspectives are also of importance as demonstrated by the need for flexibility in the functional and control-flow perspectives in the definition of KiPs, while knowledge workers themselves are part of the resource perspective and knowledge about resources can heavily influence their decisions. The languages that currently target loosely framed process (e.g., Declare, DCR graphs, GLIF, Asbru, PROforma, etc.) do not yet sufficiently address all of these perspectives together. This is the research gap that this work will try to tackle. The relative importance of the data and resource perspectives increases even more for ad hoc framed processes and ultimately dwarfs the other perspectives in the context of unframed processes.

The knowledge of process workers in KiPs guides the decision-making regarding which process variation is appropriate in a certain situation (e.g., how doctors diagnose and treat patients). The *tacit* nature of this knowledge is a typical symptom of the process being in a state of flux as the domain knowledge itself changes with time [14, 44]. The process workers cannot keep up with the complexity of the constant stream of new knowledge, which results in a situation where everyone has a different subset of the total, possibly even out-of-date, knowledge. Additionally, nobody knows exactly what the other process workers know. This tacit knowledge phenomenon is an important obstacle when attempting to accurately model these processes [48]. Stimulating and managing the knowledge conversion processes in order to externalize the tacit knowledge (i.e., linking sets of data values to certain outcomes) is an important part of improving these processes. Firstly, the explicit knowledge can be used for explaining decisions that were made [49]. Secondly, making process knowledge explicit increases the transparency of the process to all stakeholders, and hence facilitates communication of process changes or new insights as the process evolves [49]. Thirdly, making the process knowledge explicit is beneficial for training process workers. Fourthly, explicit process knowledge enables offering a more uniform service, as the knowledge workers can compare and discuss the decision logic with each other in detail, which limits the amount of divergence [50]. Lastly, processes can be optimized more efficiently and effectively because they capture the reality more closely [51].

In this chapter, the *Design Science Research* methodology [38, 39] is followed in order to design a mixed-perspective process modeling language, called *DeciClare*, that can capture information related to all four perspectives (i.e., functional, control-flow, data and resource) when modeling loosely framed KiPs, for example, in healthcare and incident management. The language was built on a declarative foundation, because of its innate support for modeling flexible process flows. DeciClare integrates several existing extensions for declarative process modeling languages as well as new solutions for yet unaddressed shortcomings (i.e., general branching of constraints, exception handling, authorization constraints and pure time and data constraints) in order to support the strongly linked perspectives of such processes. Because the different perspectives had to be integrated into one approach, DeciClare can be categorized as a mixed-perspective modeling language (this classification is further explained in Sect. 2.2).

The chapter is structured as follows. In Sect. 2.2, the related work is discussed, as well as the distinction between mixed-perspective, multi-perspective and hybrid languages. The applied research methodology is presented in Sect. 2.3. In Sect. 2.4, the problem stated in the Sect. 2.1 is translated into a set of requirements that must be met in order to adequately model loosely framed KiPs. Section 2.5 then examines each perspective in isolation. Existing modeling languages and their extensions are shown to fulfill some of these requirements, however, additional solutions are also proposed for the requirements that are not yet met. These separate solutions are then integrated into one metamodel in Sect. 2.6 for the new mixed-perspective language fulfilling all the requirements from Sect. 2.4. Next, in Sect. 2.7, the new language is evaluated by way of expert validation based on a realistic KiP. Finally, the work is concluded in Sect. 2.9 and future work opportunities are described in Sect. 2.10.

2.2   Related Work

As stated in Sect. 2.1, the languages that currently target loosely framed process (e.g., Declare and DCR graphs) do not sufficiently address all of its needs. Recently, some steps have been taken to add the support for different perspectives to Declare [22]. However, most of the extensions have been presented as separate languages. The Declare[++] language is the only extension to combine multiple aspects of the functional/control-flow perspectives with a data perspective, but it does not fully support complex decisions (i.e., no disjunctions) and lacks a resource perspective. Compared to the solution proposed in this chapter, Declare[++] is also less expressive when it comes to time concepts. Other declarative languages have recently also put more emphasis on the different perspectives of a process. Slaats et al. [52] added a data extension to DCR graphs and Guard-Stage-Milestone language [53] was introduced, which incorporates a data-centric workflow model with declarative elements for modeling life cycles of business artifacts. These languages and language extensions are, however, not enough to model some of the more complex decisions found in KiPs, because they only allow simple decision logic (i.e., no disjunctions and decisions based on only one or at most just a few data values). Their focus is still very much on the process flow itself, and less on the decision processes that govern them. As stated by Di Ciccio et al. [31], the integration of the existing extensions is considered an avenue for future work, and to our knowledge had not yet been addressed in a satisfactory manner. In this chapter, the integration of the different perspectives has been performed, and additionally, new elements have been added as to increase the expressive power of the resulting language.

2.3   Research Methodology

This chapter applies the Design Science Research methodology [38, 39] to create the metamodel (i.e., the design artifact) of a process modeling language for loosely framed KiPs. We first defined the general requirements for the design artifact (Sect. 2.4) based on literature (i.e., Req 1 and 2) and the lessons learned from the previous iteration of this design cycle (i.e., Req 3 and 4). These general requirements were subsequently translated to sets of subrequirements that define specific language constructs that needed to be supported by the design artifact. To satisfy the requirements, we identified all existing languages and language extensions from literature that support the corresponding language perspectives and analyzed which of the corresponding subrequirements could be satisfied with the ideas from the existing languages (Sect. 2.5). For the subrequirements that were not yet satisfied, we then defined custom solutions.

As evaluation (Sect. 2.7), we focused on the effectiveness of the proposed design artifact to solve the research gap that was identified in Sect. 2.1 using the Conceptual Modeling Quality Framework [54]. For this we used the arm fracture case[1], which was first introduced in van der Aalst et al. [17] and was extended in Mertens et al. [55] through interviews with a practicing surgeon. In this work, an expert panel of four medical practitioners with a real-life connection to the case (i.e., purposive sampling) was asked to evaluate the design artifact based on the case: an experienced general surgeon, an experienced orthopedic surgeon, an orthopedic surgeon in training (intern) and an experienced emergency nurse. By using practitioners that take on different roles in the process, we tried to get different viewpoints on the same case. The surgeons could validate/provide the medical diagnosis and treatment knowledge, the nurse could validate/provide the more practical knowledge on what happens starting from when the patient enters the emergency room and the intern the could validate/provide the academic knowledge as he was taught during his education. This should result in a more complete picture, with the maximum of variance in the type of knowledge that would need to be represented.

Design Science research is an iterative process [38] and this work presents our second iteration of the subject. This chapter should not be considered an extension of the previous iteration [55], but it rather restarts from scratch while incorporating the lessons learned from the previous iteration. Firstly, this work abandons the ambition to propose both an abstract and a concrete syntax for the language in one cycle. As stated by Moody [56], both require a different approach and evaluation (i.e., semantic versus cognitive). Consequently, it is better to split them in two separate research steps so that each can be performed in greater depth and with a separate evaluation. This work presents the first part of the research project: the development of an abstract syntax for a modeling language that targets loosely framed KiPs. An implementation of this abstract syntax in the form of an Ecore model is the resulting design science artifact. Secondly, this work starts from a better theoretical foundation in the form of specific requirements for the language based on the needs of the targeted processes. This allowed for a more thorough analysis of the existing solutions (i.e., mostly extensions of declarative process modeling languages) as well as to identify remaining shortcomings. The resulting requirements thus served as a blueprint for designing the envisioned language. Lastly, an evaluation of the effectiveness of the proposed language by way of interviews with domain experts was also added.

2.4 Language Requirements

The *main goal* of this chapter is the development of a process modeling language that allows for the functional, control-flow, resource and data perspectives of loosely

---

[1]Note that the arm fracture case was only used during the evaluation phase. It was only during the writing of the paper that we decided to introduce the case earlier in the paper, so we could use it to illustrate the subrequirements and provide examples throughout the paper

framed KiPs to be modeled in an integrated manner. These perspectives should not be treated in isolation, because the different perspectives are naturally intertwined. For instance, the required execution of an activity (i.e., functional/control-flow perspectives) could tie up certain resources thereby impacting the general resource availabilities (i.e., resource perspective), while the activity itself could use and produce certain data elements (i.e., data perspective). Alternatively, the unavailability of a resource (i.e., resource perspective) can result in the direct unavailability of an activity that requires the resource for its execution (i.e., functional/control-flow perspectives) and trigger decisions on how to respond to this unavailability (i.e., data perspective). Lastly, changing a data value (i.e., data perspective) could result in different activities needing to be executed (i.e., functional/control-flow perspectives) and adjusted resources availabilities (i.e., resource perspective). These domino effects between the perspectives are a common feature in many processes, but the relative prominence of all four of the perspectives in loosely framed KiPs (see Sect. 2.1) increases the need to capture these effects in the process models. Therefore, the developed process modeling language will have to be of a mixed-perspective nature (see Sect. 2.2) in order to integrate the different perspectives into one combined modeling technique.

The main goal can be translated into *five subgoals*: four subgoals expressing the need to support each of the perspectives and one additional subgoal for the integration of the different perspectives. These general subgoals can be operationalized to specific requirements for the modeling language by taking into account the properties and needs of loosely framed KiPs. There is one less requirement than there are subgoals, because the first requirement applies for both the functional and control-flow perspectives of the process. In the remainder of this section, these four requirements are presented and explained.

Req 1: The language must support 'flexibility by design'

The first requirement relates to the *functional* and *control-flow* perspectives. Loosely framed processes allow many different arrangements of their activities, leading to a large variety of process variations being valid [6, 18]. For example, take the diagnosis of a patient in an oncology department. The doctor can do any number of tests selected from a battery of possible tests to check whether or not the patient has cancer, and if so, determine the type, the size, the aggressiveness and the stage of the cancer. There are many different sequences in which these tests can be done, but some sequences can or cannot occur depending on certain prerequisite conditions specific to each process instance. To model such highly-dynamic, human-centric, knowledge-intensive and non-standardized processes, a language is needed that supports the flexibility to model these variations and defers the choice for a certain variation to the run-time execution [16]. This type of flexibility is called *flexibility by design* [20]. Flexibility by design thus implies that many alternative process variations are designed into the process model implicitly, allowing the choice of a suitable variation to be made at run-time for each individual process instance.

> **Req 2: The language must offer support for modeling complex decisions**

The 'knowledge' in KiPs alludes to the implicit or explicit knowledge needed by the process workers to execute the process. Let us retake the example from the oncology department from the previous paragraph and suppose that the doctor has determined that the patient has a brain stem tumor. There are several ways for the process to proceed and, obviously, the process variation to follow is not chosen at random. To learn the type of cancer cells one would normally perform a biopsy, but, because of the location of the tumor, patient safety regulations state that this goes out the window. The doctor would have to resort to using an MRI, CT and/or some other imaging test to proceed. This is an example of a rather simple rule using process relevant data, in this case data generated during one or more previous activities, followed by a decision on how to proceed. KiPs are governed by many rules and/or decisions processes [6, 21] and insight into these decisions is at least as important as what activities are available for execution, so support for decision modeling should be included in modeling language proposed in this work. Because, at its core, decision modeling is nothing more than linking data values or combinations of data values to outcomes, this comes down to incorporating a *data* perspective into the language. The knowledge of a process is represented by the combination of specific data values and outcomes used in its decision-making. Typically, decisions that govern the process execution of KiPs have a high perceived complexity [6]. Some contributing factors to the decision complexity are the number of data values and data value aggregations used, the number of data sources and the number of decision conditions as well as their interrelations. The data perspective of the language thus needs to offer support for modeling complex decisions that guide process execution.

> **Req 3: The language needs to allow reasoning about resources**

Resources play a vital role in loosely framed KiPs. More often than not, the execution of certain activities from the functional and control-flow perspectives depends on the availability of certain resources and those resources have certain properties expressed in data values (e.g., availability, speed, cost, quality, etc.) that influence the decisions in the data perspective of the process model. So, the modeling language needs to incorporate some form of *resource* perspective to help paint a complete picture of the process and its resources. For example, resources need to be taken into account to make the models executable, to allow a thorough analysis of the process, to offer meaningful guidance to process workers and to facilitate simulation and optimization techniques.

> **Req 4: The language must define a clear link between the different perspectives while carefully considering the domain appropriateness**

Finally, the last requirement relates the previous three requirements. As stated at the start of this section, the four perspectives are closely linked. These relationships are complementary in most cases, however, overlaps exist. The functional/control-flow and data perspectives have an innate overlap in expressive power. For example, stating that activity B must be executed after activity A can, in theory, be represented as a part of either perspective. In the control-flow perspective it would result in a temporal relation between the two activities, while in the data perspective it would be a decision with the execution of activity A (= a fact, hence data) as condition and the execution of activity B as an outcome. This is an example of construct redundancy [57], signaling that there exist multiple ways to represent the same ontological concept in a language. According to [58] the truthfulness of a modeling language with respect to the domain depends on the degree of isomorphism between the meta-model of the language and the domain conceptualization, also referred to as the *domain appropriateness*. Construct redundancy, excess and overload are all properties that serve as telltale signs of a misalignment of the domain appropriateness of a language. As a consequence, the way in which the four perspectives are linked and complement each other should be carefully considered.

2.5 Designing the Perspectives

In this section a standalone metamodel for each of the perspectives, required by *requirements 1, 2 and 3* from the previous section, will be developed. In Sect. 2.6, we integrate these metamodels to also fulfil requirement 4. The concepts used in this section are defined on a rather abstract level to allow them to apply to a broad range of cases, which can make the link with real-life needs unclear. Therefore, a case description of realistic KiP will first be introduced to serve as a source of examples to demonstrate the practical relevance of the concepts used. The same case will also be used in Sect. 2.7 to evaluate the proposed language.

2.5.1 The Arm Fracture Case

As a practical example of a KiP, the realistic healthcare process of diagnosing and treating patients with suspected arm fractures created in Mertens et al. [55] will be used (see Appendix A for a full description). This is not an isolated process in real-life, but rather a part of the general process spanning the emergency and orthopedic departments of a hospital. For this reason, we will use the term 'realistic' instead of 'real-life' to indicate the difference between the artificially reduced scope of the case compared to the even more complex real-life case. The scope of arm fracture case is limited to patients with one or more suspected fractures in his or her fingers, hands, wrists, forearms, upper arms, shoulders, and/or collarbones. The activities related to the admission, diagnosis and treatment phases are included (see Table 2.1).

Table 2.1 The activities used in the arm fracture case

Admission	Register patient, Unregister patient
Diagnosis	Take medical history of patient, Clinical examination of patient, Doctor consultation, Take X-ray, Take CT scan, Apply intra-compartmental pressure monitor
Treatment	Prescribe NSAID painkillers, Prescribe SAID painkillers, Prescribe anticoagulants, Prescribe stomach protecting drug, Prescribe rest (= no treatment), Apply ice, Apply cast, Remove cast, Apply splint, Apply sling, Apply fixation, Remove fixation, Apply bandage, Apply figure of eight bandage, Perform surgery, Let patient rest, Stay in patient room

In the remainder of this section, examples from this case will be used where possible. Just a few types of modeling concepts do not occur in this case. So, for these concepts examples from other healthcare processes will be used.

2.5.2 Declare as a Foundation

Support for the flexibility by design principle (*requirement 1*) in the functional and control-flow perspectives can be achieved in multiple ways. In BPM there are two major modeling approaches: *imperative* and *declarative* process modeling [16, 59]. Process modeling languages like BPMN [60] and Petri nets [61, 62] are examples of imperative modeling languages (also known as procedural languages). These techniques can be described, in essence, as inside-out approaches to modeling because they describe exactly what the allowed behavior during process execution is (i.e., they provide an enumeration of all valid process variations) [17]. Consequently, imperative process modeling languages are well suited to model tightly framed processes as for such processes only a limited number of process variations need to be modeled. Declarative process modeling languages like Declare [22] and DCR graphs [23] take the opposite viewpoint with an outside-in approach. Declarative languages describe the rules and constraints by which the process must abide [16]. The unwanted process variations are prohibited based on these rules and constraints, while all other variations are allowed without explicitly having to enumerate all valid variations [17].

Although imperative process modeling languages can also support the flexibility by design principle, declarative process modeling languages are better suited for modeling loosely framed processes as they do not require enumerating the potentially large number of valid process variations [18]. Generally, given the large number of allowed process variations in loosely framed processes, less effort will be required to describe the properties that make variations valid or invalid compared to enumerating all the valid process variations explicitly like imperative languages [7, 16].

The Declare modeling language will be used as the foundation of our language, since it is currently one of the most popular and comprehensive declarative process modeling languages and it has many available extensions. Mulyar et al. [63] has also shown that this language enables the representation of typical clinical guidelines, which are part of many loosely framed KiPs in healthcare. Declare is based on Linear Temporal Logic (LTL) [17, 22] and allows for process models to be defined in terms of activities and constraints spanning these activities. The process environment is specified in terms of what is necessary and what is not allowed (i.e., rules expressing the modal verb 'must' and 'must not'), restricting the possible process executions. Contrary to other declarative languages like DCR Graphs and BPCN [64], Declare also supports guidelines (referred to as optional constraints). Such constraints offer guidance (i.e., rules expressing the modal verbs 'should' and 'ought to'), while their soft character ensures flexibility is maintained (i.e., it is not necessary to enforce them) [16].

There are three main groups of Declare constraint templates (i.e., templates that can be used to create actual constraints in Declare models) defined in the description of the Declare language [22]:

Existence constraints: unary constraints predicating the allowed or mandatory amount of executions of an activity (e.g., existence(3, A) stating that activity A must be executed at least 3 times).

- Choice constraints: n-ary constraints expressing a choice between activities from a given set (e.g., choice(2, [A, B, C]) stating that at least 2 distinct activities among A, B and C must be executed).
- Relation constraints: binary constraints enforcing a relation between two activities (e.g., response(A, B) stating that if A is executed, then B must be executed at any time after A). Also negative versions of these relation constraints exist (e.g., responded_absence(A, B) stating that if A is executed, then B can never be executed).

In the arm fracture case, for example, the general flow of the process states that a doctor can choose from several activities to reach a diagnosis and a wide range of possible treatments activities. However, an X-ray should be taken in almost every case (we will ignore the exception of life-threatening cases for now), immediately followed by a consultation with the patient to discuss the results. Imperative modeling language would require the explicit enumeration of every valid sequence of diagnosis and treatment steps. For example, a variation needs to be defined for when the doctor decides on a treatment consisting of an X-ray, a consultation, a prescription for painkillers and the application of a sling. But it should also be possible to give the patient the painkillers and/or sling before taking the X-ray. So even for this simple case, which does not even take into account the any prior steps, it will result in six variations depending on the order of these steps. Declare allows this to be modeled with just two constraints: *existence(1, Take X-ray)* and *chain_response(Take X-ray, Doctor consultation)*. All the variations that do not violate these constraints are implicitly allowed.

We created a metamodel of the Declare language (Fig. 2.1), because a complete metamodel of Declare is not available in literature. This metamodel is based on a partial metamodel of the Declare language [65] and the implicit metamodel of the

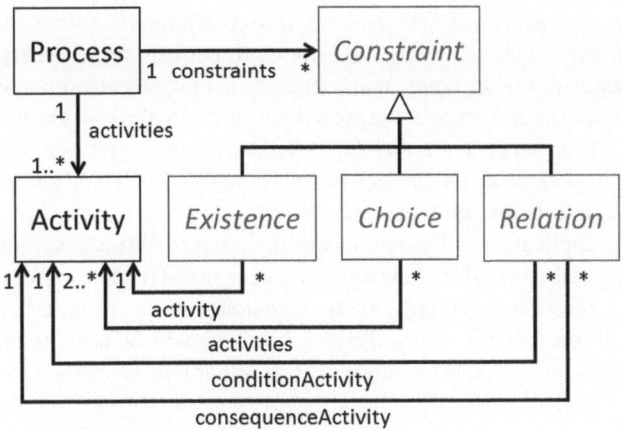

Fig. 2.1 The metamodel of the Declare language

concrete syntax proposed for the language [22] and the corresponding modeling tool[2]. The constraint templates themselves have been omitted from the metamodel to maintain a manageable overview and will be presented later on. Having an explicit metamodel for a modeling language is important as it represents the core concepts of the language and their relationships. This prevents possible ambiguity, which can make a language more difficult to use. It is also a necessary step to be able to correctly integrate new elements into a language and for any kind of tool support to be developed.

The metamodel in Fig. 2.1 captures the Declare language as it has been used in most research, with the existence and choice templates largely corresponding to the functional perspective and the relation templates to the control-flow perspective. However, there is one change that could already be made. This entails using events in addition to activities, similar to how this was proposed in [66]. Pesic [22] defines the Declare constraint templates using activities as parameters. However, in the partial metamodel proposed in Bernardi et al. [65] constraints are actually already linked with events as opposed to activities. This ambiguity is probably due to the use of events in the underlying LTL definitions for each of the templates in [22] and could have been avoided by providing an explicit metamodel of the language. The effect of allowing the templates to use event parameters is that it allows for much more fine-grained control when it comes to the expressive power of the constraints. Activities have a life cycle consisting of a start, end and cancellation event, mirroring the LTL definitions in Pesic [22]. For example, stating that a physical examination cannot be performed before the doctor or nurse has already started asking the patient questions about his/her medical history, can now be expressed with a precedence

---

[2]http://www.win.tue.nl/declare/

constraint: *precedence(start(Take medical history of patient), start(Clinical examination of patient))*. This still leaves the option to perform these activities simultaneously or sequentially. In comparison, the original precedence template is always assumed to relate the end event of the preceding activity to the start event of the subsequent activity (i.e., *precedence(end(Take medical history of patient), start(Clinical examination of patient)))*. Other declarative languages like DCR graphs also work on the level of events for similar reasons [52].

During the application of Declare in specific process contexts, several shortcomings of the original scope of the language have been noted (e.g., resources, time, etc.). In response to these shortcomings, many standalone extensions have been proposed for Declare in the past few years. These extensions will be used as inspiration or starting point for the proposed solutions for the other requirements.

2.5.3 Extending the Functional and Control-Flow Perspectives

With Declare as the foundation to build on, the match between its expressive power concerning the functional and control-flow perspectives and the needs of loosely framed KiPs can be analyzed. We specified a set of seven rule patterns that typically occur in this type of process based on the overview of rule patterns in Caron et al. [67] (i.e., A, B and C) and additional insights obtained from studying several loosely-framed processes in healthcare organizations (i.e., D, E, F and G). Each pattern can entail multiple constraints that differ in effect but are all related to a same underlying concept. These rule patterns, accompanied by an example of such a constraint in healthcare diagnosis and treatment processes, are presented in Table 2.2.

Table 2.2 Seven typical rule patterns for flexible and KiPs

	Rule pattern	Example
A	*Cardinalities*	A patient must be registered exactly once
B	*Coexistence*	At least two of the following treatments will be administered: surgery, a cast, a fixation, bandages and painkillers
C	*Temporal relationships*	If a patient has had surgery, then he will receive anticoagulants afterwards
D	*Negative relationships*	NSAID and SAID painkillers should not be administered simultaneously
E	*n-ary relationships*	Taking a CT or X-ray scan must be followed by a consultation with a doctor
F	*Exception handling*	If a patient has an adverse reaction to the anesthesia causing the doctors to abandon the rest of the surgery, this is followed by a consultation to determine what needs to happen next
G	*Guidelines*	Directly after surgery, the responsible doctor should visit the patient to explain what was done and what is next (i.e., a consultation)

The available Declare templates can immediately fulfil several rule patterns. The existence templates of Declare can enforce the cardinalities of rule pattern *A* (for the example from Table 2.2: *existence(1, start(Register patient)) and absence(1, start(Register patient)))*. Rule pattern *B* can be fulfilled with the choice and responded existence templates *A* (for the example from Table 2.2: *choice(1, start(Perform surgery), start(Apply cast), start(Apply fixation), start(Apply bandage), start(Prescribe painkillers)))*. Constraints belonging to rule patterns *C* and *D* can be expressed by using the relation templates (for the example from Table 2.2: *response(end(Perform surgery), start(Prescribe anticoagulants))* and *not_chain_succession(end(Prescribe NSAID), start(Prescribe SAID)))*. And lastly, Declare also supports optional constraints, which can be used to model the guidelines of rule pattern *G* (for the example from Table 2.2: *optional response(end(Perform surgery), start(Doctor consultation)))*. However, support for rule patterns *E* and *F* is lacking, and thus, needs to be addressed.

Before addressing the unsupported rule patterns, we will make a small change to the choice templates that were used to support rule pattern *B*. The exclusive choice template is replaced by the *AtMostChoice* template (the normal choice template will also be renamed to *AtLeastChoice*, see Table 2.7). The exclusive choice template states that exactly the given number of activities from the given set must be executed. Keeping in mind that the normal choice template expresses the same thing but with the 'exactly' replaced by 'at least', it seems strange to ignore that the 'exactly' can also be replaced by a template expressing 'at most'. Similar to the other templates of the existence type, the 'exactly' is merely a combination of an 'at least' and an 'at most' constraint with the same bound and activities. Therefore, adding the AtMostChoice template results in an increase of the expressive power and symmetry of the constraint templates.

Rule pattern *E* is the first unsupported rule pattern that will be discussed, as this entails a fundamental change to the Declare definitions. It conveys the need to express the constraints with more than the predefined number of connected elements. In the original definitions of the Declare constraint templates, constraints are connected to one (i.e., existence, with the exception of the choice templates) or two activities (i.e., relation) each. By *branching* the constraint templates, each connected element is replaced by a non-empty set of connected elements (e.g., *response([A and B], [C or D or E])*). Pesic [22] already described this as a possible extension of Declare, while later work elaborated further on the subject of branching. Montali [66] provided a definition for branching relation templates, while the TBDeclare extension [31] focusses on branching of the consequence side (sometimes referred to as the target side) of relation templates. The broadest definition of branching will be used, and thus, allow branching for all constraint templates. Although the definitions in the above-mentioned extensions always use an inclusive disjunctive interpretation of the branched parameters, DeciClare will sometimes also allow conjunctions and represent them as logical expressions. The introduction of branching impacts the templates in different ways:

The original definitions of the choice templates are, in a sense, already branched according to the interpretation of a disjunction. This will be expanded with conjunctions. For example, the choice template (later referred to as the AtLeastChoice template) can be used to specify that at least one out of the three following options must be executed: w or x or (y and z). This constraint would allow event traces like *[w], [x], [y, z], [w, x, y]...*, but not *[y], [z], [y, y]...*

The absence template (later referred to as the AtMost template) now supports both the inclusive disjunction and the logical conjunction for its logical expressions. For example, consider an event trace of *[x, x, x, z, y, y]*. It is correct to state that x *or* y occur at most 5 times (i.e., *AtMost([x or y], 5)*), corresponding to the sum of the occurrences of x and the occurrences of y being at most 5. On the other hand, it is correct to state that x *and* y occur at most 2 times (i.e., *AtMost([x and y], 2)*), corresponding to the minimum number of occurrences of x and y separately being at most 2. This is because at most 2 (x, y)-pairs can be found in the trace.

For the existence template (AtLeast) similar logic applies for the disjunction. However, the conjunction is not supported because, for example, requiring at least a certain number of occurrences of (x, y)-pairs is equivalent to requiring x and y to separately occur at least that many times (i.e., two separate AtLeast-constraints). To represent this in one statement could be useful for a concrete syntax, but in the metamodel of the language this will be avoided because this is syntactic sugar (see Sect. 2.6.3).

The relation templates, as presented in Montali [66], support the inclusive disjunction. But this can also be further extended to include the expression of logical conjunctions. For example, consider a response constraint *Response([x or [y and z]], [w])*. This expresses that when event x has been executed or both events y and z have been executed, event w eventually needs to be executed. The example used in Table 2.2 can now be modeled as *Response([end(Take CT scan) or end(Take X-ray)], [start(Doctor consultation)])*.

Rule pattern *F* corresponds to exception handling constraints. It can be supported by introducing a *failure event*. Similar to the cancellation event, it marks an alternative ending of the execution of the corresponding activity, although this time not in a user-driven fashion (e.g., due to a change of heart by the patient). The constraint templates can now be used to specify what must happen when failure occurs. However, some combinations make little or no sense (e.g., the end event of activity A must be responded by the failure of activity B), while others are just hard to enforce (e.g., the failure of activity A can occur no more than once). Our suggestion would be to use the event only in combination with the responded existence, response and precedence templates (including their variations) with the additional limitation that it cannot be included in the condition parameter connected to the precedence templates, nor in the consequence parameter connected to the other templates. For instance, the failure event can be used in a ChainResponse constraint to express that if an MRI scan fails because the patient had unexpected metal items in his/her body (e.g., hip replacement), then immediate surgery must be performed to repair the damage done by the MRI magnet. The example used in Table 2.2 can now be modeled as *ChainResponse([failure(Perform surgery)], [start(Doctor consultation)])*.

To allow for a shorter notation of the constraints, we will introduce a default event interpretation of an activity in a constraint. The start event of the activity will be the default interpretation for the existence and choice templates when only the activity name is used in the template. For example, *AtLeast([start(Register patient)], 1)* is the same as *AtLeast([Register patient], 1)*. For the relation templates, we will use the end event as the default interpretation for the condition side and the start event for the consequence side. For example, *Response([end(Perform surgery)], [start(Apply cast)])* is the same as *Response([Perform surgery], [Apply cast])*. Note that this means that the default interpretation of the previous example does not state that the cast must be successfully applied, just that the activity of applying the cast must be started. This leaves room for exception handling behavior to be specified, as the successful execution of an activity cannot be guaranteed.

2.5.4 Adding a Notion of Time-Awareness to the Constraint Templates

Dadam et al. [68] stated that the minimal and maximal time before, after and between activities is an important aspect in many loosely framed processes. The rule patterns presented in Table 2.2 do not deal with time as an explicit concept, as they largely coincide with expressive power of the original Declare language. Caron et al. [67] also proposed two more rule patterns that deal with time as a concept (*T1* and *T2* in Table 2.3). Additionally, Lanz et al. [69] have suggested a set of time patterns for supporting *time-awareness* in process-aware information systems based on empirical evidence from case studies (*T3-T7* in Table 2.3). Some of the time patterns suggested

Table 2.3 Seven time patterns to complement the control-flow perspectives

	Time pattern	Example
T1	*Time-oriented existence*	The triage must be started within 5 min of the process start
T2	*Time-oriented relationships*	After surgery for a displaced or unstable fracture of the leg, a cast is applied. This cast cannot be removed within the first 10 weeks after surgery
T3	*Lag between two activities*	The time between on the one side removing a cast and having done an X-ray and on the other side starting a doctor consultation, should be at most 15 min
T4	*Durations*	The triage should not exceed 10 min
T5	*Lag between arbitrary events*	The time between the start of the triage and the start of an examination by a doctor should not exceed 3 min for patients with a high-risk level
T6	*Schedule restricted elements*	Lab tests can be requested on Mondays between 8 am and 5 pm
T7	*Cyclic elements*	Patients with medium risk level should be checked every hour

in Lanz et al. have been omitted, because they do not apply in the context of loosely-framed KiPs or are redundant as a result of other patterns presented throughout this chapter.

Declare supports an implicit idea of time (e.g., sequencing), but it lacks the support for *metric time* as is needed to satisfy the rule patterns in Table 2.3. However, the idea of supporting metric time in Declare is not new. [66, 70, 71] have all identified a need for constraint templates using time units. To solve this, a reformulation of Declare, called Timed Declare, was proposed in *Metric Temporal Logic* (MTL) that adds the option to express time units [71]. As a result, new versions of all Declare templates were defined. For example, the timed response template can express that a doctor consultation needs to take place at some point in time, t_1, after the taking an X-ray at t_0, with $t_1 \in [\ t_0 + a, t_0 + b\ ]$. The inclusion or exclusion of the boundaries of the interval can be specified in the template using the parameters a and b which are expressed in time units (b is allowed to be ∞). When a and b respectively equal 0 and ∞, the formula collapses to the original definition of the response constraints of Declare. These MTL-definitions of the templates will be used instead of the original LTL-definitions as a starting point for our DeciClare language, because this reformulation increases the expressive power of Declare with a notion of time-awareness.

The time parameters of the Timed Declare constraint templates add a notion of time to the constraint templates that is sufficient to satisfy time patterns *T1* (for the example from Table 2.3: *AtLeast([Triage], 1, 0, 5 min)*) and *T2* (for the example from Table 2.3: *NotResponse([Perform surgery], [Remove cast], 0, 10weeks)*). However, the other time patterns are not supported yet. *T3*, *T4* and *T5* can be treated jointly as the language already works on the granularity level of events. The time between two activities (*T3*) is defined as the time between the end event of the first activity and the start event of the second activity. *T5* generalizes this to the time between any two events of the process. This means that it also covers the duration of an activity (*T4*), because the duration is equal to the time between the start and end event of the activity. As a result, two new time constraints will be defined to add support for these three patterns: *AtLeastLag* and *AtMostLag*. These constraint templates have two logical expressions using events (inclusive disjunction and conjunction) as input parameters and express that the time between the satisfaction of the first expression and the second expression can be no less or no more, respectively, than a given limit expressed in time units (for the example from Table 2.3: *AtMostLag([end(Remove cast) and end(Take X-ray)], [start(Doctor consultation))], 15 min)*). The sixth time pattern (*T6*) makes it possible to express that certain activities are only available for execution according to a certain schedule. This can be generalized to also include expressing that certain activities are unavailable for execution according to a schedule (e.g., maintenance). For this, another two constraints are added: *EventAvailabilitySchedule* and *EventUnavailabilitySchedule*. Their parameters are a logical expression using events (inclusive disjunction) and a schedule. A schedule is a set of statements that take on the following form '(mandatory) every *[periodic point in time]*, (optional) between *[two smaller periodic points in time]*'. The example from Table 2.3 would now be modeled as *EventAvailabilitySchedule([Lab tests], [every Monday between 8 am and 5 pm])*. The last time pattern (*T7*) enables the use of cyclic elements in the

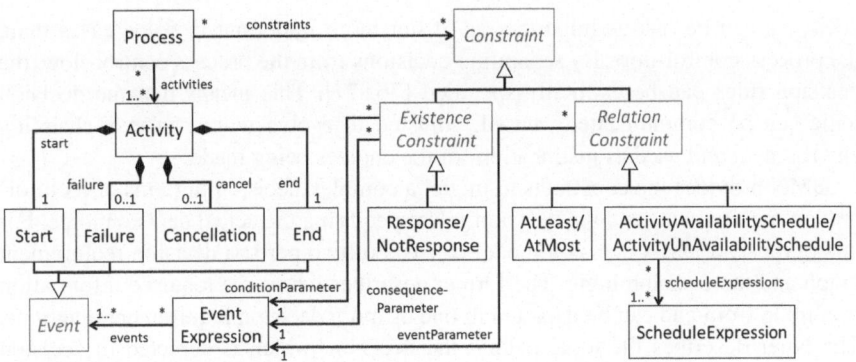

Fig. 2.2 The metamodel of the functional (left) and control-flow (right) perspectives

process. Where the Timed Declare definitions can be used to specify that an activity or event must be executed a certain number of times within a certain time interval, *T7* adds to option to specify the time lag between the different executions. This can also be modeled with the first two new time constraint templates (i.e., *AtLeastLag* and *AtMostLag*), and so, requires no additional changes.

Taking all of the changes from this subsection and the previous one into account produces the extended Timed and Branched Declare metamodel in Fig. 2.2. This represents the functional and control-flow perspectives in response to *requirement 1*. Note that the left side of the metamodel corresponds with the functional perspective and the right side with the control-flow perspective of DeciClare.

2.5.5   Supporting the Data Perspective

Until recently, no attempt had been made to support the data perspective in declarative languages [72]. The languages lacked the expressive power to adequately model the (tacit) knowledge that governs the execution of loosely framed and KiPs [55, 73]. Recent publications [52, 74, 75] have proposed extensions that add some data-awareness to the main declarative languages, including Declare. Even though this is a good start, none of the proposed extensions contain all of the elements needed to offer a complete solution for *requirement 2*. The extensions allow for data to be linked to constraints of the control-flow perspective (cf. Sect. 2.6.1), but they do not sufficiently specify the data perspective itself (e.g., Which data attributes are there? When are they assigned/changed? etc.).

The decision modeling standard from the OMG group [49], *Decision Model and Notation (DMN)*, served as inspiration during the formulation of a metamodel for the Declare data perspective. The primary goal of DMN is to provide a common notation for decision logic that can be understood by business users, business analysts and technical developers. This new standard is a response to the rising awareness that decisions can be just as important as, if not more important in some cases than, the process control-flow. By separating decisions from the process control-flow, the decision rules can be explicitly specified [76, 77]. This means that the decision logic can be communicated, reused, adjusted to evolve within an ever-changing environment and used as justification for the choices being made.

DMN provides the constructs to model a complex decision in terms of its information requirements and the decision rules specifying the actual decision logic. For this purpose, a DMN decision model consists of two parts: a decision requirement graph and the decision logic. The former describes where the required information is coming from and can be depicted in one or more decision requirement diagrams. The latter describes the logic behind the decision, which is depicted in decision tables [78]. Decision tables were chosen as the only representation of decision logic currently supported by DMN, because they are very popular and easy to understand. The current minimal scope of DMN will be expanded to include other representations (e.g., decision trees) and allow for references to other types of models (e.g., SBVR) in the future as the standard evolves [79]. The standard also describes its link to the popular imperative process modeling language BPMN explicitly through the Decision Task, but it positions itself as a separate perspective usable in other contexts as well [49]. However, it is unclear how it can be used in combination with other languages, including declarative process modeling languages.

For the purpose of this work, the focus will only be on the underlying concepts used by DMN to model decisions. The same concepts will be integrated in our metamodel, as to keep the option open to also use the same visual notations in future research. The upper half of a decision table specifies the possible combinations of conditions, while the bottom half contains the actions to be taken (i.e., outcomes). This allows for complex decision logic to be modeled in one decision table or be spread over multiple tables. shows the metamodel for decision tables. A metamodel of the decision requirement graphs, which can be used to specify where the data values in the decision tables come from as well as the relations between decision tables, has been omitted as these graphs are non-essential for representing the actual decision logic and do not require integration into the other perspectives.

The decision rules in Fig. 2.3 use unary tests as input entries. In turn, these tests use the values of data attributes to return a Boolean answer (e.g., patient gender = 'female'). Adding the concepts of a simple data model to Fig. 2.3 results in Fig. 2.4. A data record (e.g., patient file), possibly containing multiple sub records (e.g., medical

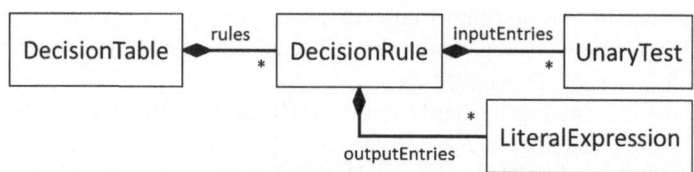

Fig. 2.3 The metamodel of the DMN language for specifying decision logic (based on Figure 51 from [49])

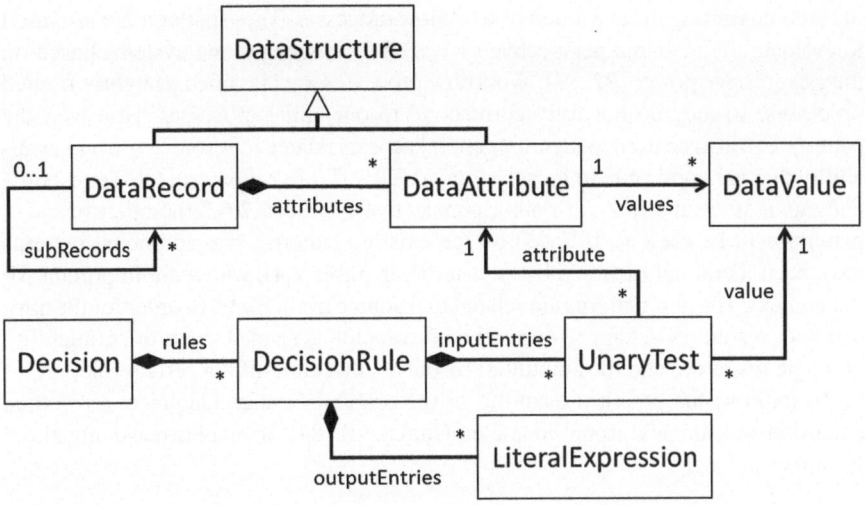

Fig. 2.4 The metamodel of the proposed data extension

history), consists of a set of data attributes (e.g., patient allergies), which each have one or more values connected to them (e.g., allergies = {'penicillin', 'peanuts'}). The unary tests are now Boolean statements using these values (e.g., 'the patient has an allergy to penicillin?').

Finally, a last remark on how the decisions themselves are to be modeled in Deci-Clare. The principles of imperative and declarative modeling can, in a sense, also be applied to decision logic. Imperative decision logic could correspond to decisions that have explicit outcomes for all possible combinations of the conditions (i.e., satisfy completeness property). Contrarily, a declarative description of decision logic could correspond to decisions that do not fulfill this property. These decisions only describe the outcomes for a subset of all the possible combinations of conditions, leaving the rest unspecified. For example, a decision based on one Boolean data attribute is specified completely (i.e., imperatively) if separate actions are defined for when the data value equals 'True' and when the data value equals 'False'. A declarative decision based on one Boolean data attribute specifies an action for one of the data values and leaves the other one unspecified. This follows the over- and underspecification tendencies of, respectively, the imperative and declarative way of thinking. As Deci-Clare takes on a declarative viewpoint, it follows that the specification of decision logic will also use this viewpoint.

2.5.6 Supporting the Resource Perspective

The resource patterns defined in [10, 80, 81] can be used as inspiration for adding an resource perspective to the language (*requirement 3*). The patterns show typical use of resources during the execution of workflow processes. These patterns are also used to evaluate the resource perspective of workflow languages and systems based on their expressive power [82, 83]. Workflow processes are classified as tightly framed processes, so they do not fully correspond to our target processes. However, the patterns can also be used to identify general aspects related to resource use and availability that are applicable to loosely framed KiPs. Table 2.4 presents those resource patterns that are not linked to other perspectives, in Sect. 2.6.2 the other resource patterns will be presented. Based on the existing patterns, two additional patterns have been identified (denoted by an asterisk in Table 2.4), which are important for our context. The new patterns are related to resource availability. In order for the allocation of resources to happen correctly, information is needed about the availability of single resources and the amount of resources that can fulfill a certain role.

To improve the practical usability of the original Declare language, a resource extension was already proposed, called ConDec-R [84]. It enables reasoning about resources in Declare:

- Defining resources and the number of available instances of each resource type
- For each activity, linking the resource(s) required for its execution
- For each activity, adding estimates of its duration, cost or any other property

As there is again no metamodel publicly available, a metamodel was created based on the proposed semantics of Jiménez-Ramírez and Barba (Fig. 2.5). The ConDec-R extension does not clearly define what types of resources are included. Based on the example usage of the language in Jiménez-Ramírez and Barba, resource reasoning

Table 2.4 Three resource patterns relevant to flexible and KiPs

	Resource pattern	Example
R1	Direct availability*	The hospital has two operating rooms (no.1 and no.2) and operating room no.1 is only available on Wednesdays between 8 am and 11 am
R2	Role-based availability*	The hospital has 20 available receptionists
R3	Simultaneous execution	A recovery room can simultaneously handle up to 10 patients

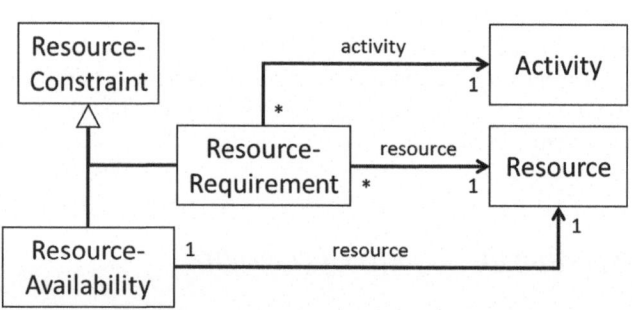

Fig. 2.5 The metamodel of the resource extension of the ConDec-R language

capabilities were added with non-human resources in mind. However, the definition of the resource-element in the metamodel can be expanded to also include human resources. Note that the metamodel already links Resource to Activity, and thus provides a link between the resource and functional/control-flow perspectives. This part of the metamodel will be discussed in Sect. 2.6.2.

In terms of the resource patterns of Table 2.4, this metamodel directly satisfies pattern *R2*. The example from Table 2.4 can be modeled as *ResourceAvailability(Receptionist, 20)*. However, that metamodel cannot express, for example, that the sum of available doctors and nurses is five (independent of the actual distribution). By introducing branched resource constraint templates, similar to the control-flow constraint templates, this can be modeled as *ResourceAvailability([Doctor and Nurse], 5)*. Additionally, some extra flexibility can be added by specifying a lower and upper bound similar to the existence templates, instead of specifying the exact number of available instances of a resource. Branched resource constraint templates *AtLeastAvailable* and *AtMostAvailable* have been added, which have a logical expression using resources (inclusive disjunction), a lower or upper bound and two time bounds as parameters. For example, *AtLeastAvailable([Doctor and Nurse], 5, 0, ∞)* expresses that the sum of available doctors and nurses at any time during the process must be at least five. Although it is not directly required by the resources patterns, resource versions of the *ResourceAvailabilitySchedule* and *ResourceUnavailabilitySchedule* templates (*T6*) have also been added. The reasons for some activities to be (un-)available according to a certain schedule typically directly originates from the availability of a certain required resource according to the same or similar schedule. A typical example of this would be lab tests. Activities like performing blood and DNA testing rely on the availability of the lab for their execution. By adding these templates, the models can represent the reason for this (un-)availability more precisely (i.e., Perform DNA test requires a lab and *ResourceAvailabilitySchedule([Lab], [every Tuesday between 11 am and 4 pm and every Friday between 9 am and 6 pm])*).

Support for the direct availability of resources (*R1*), for example stating that operating room no.1 is only available on Tuesdays between 8 and 11 a.m., can be added by allowing a resource to be either a *direct resource* (e.g., dr. Gregory House or operating room no.1) or a *resource role* (e.g., orthopedic surgeon or operating room). A direct resource then of course can be part of a resource role (e.g., operating rooms no.1 and no.2 can satisfy the role of operating room: *Operating room(operating room no.1, operating room no.2)*). By allowing the resources roles to be further specialized, even more elaborate reasoning about resources is made possible (e.g., a doctor can have a specialization of neurosurgeon).

The last unsupported resource pattern deals with resources that can handle multiple resource allocations simultaneously (*R3*). This can be implemented by introducing one last constraint template: *SimultaneousCapacity*. It has a resource and an integer as input, combined with the standard two time parameters. The example from Table 2.4 can now be expressed as follows: *SimultaneousCapacity([Recovery room], 10, 0, ∞)*.

Integrating the solutions for the metamodel of the resource perspective, results in the metamodel presented in Fig. 2.6.

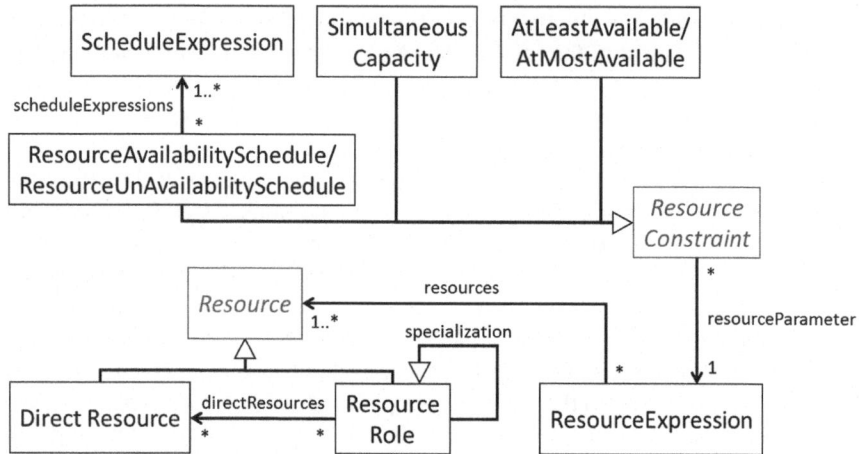

Fig. 2.6 The metamodel of the proposed resource extension

2.6   Integrating the Perspectives

The previous section proposed extensions for Declare resulting in three standalone metamodels, enabling the functional/control-flow, data and resource perspectives of a process to be represented. These metamodels are merely partial solutions to *requirements 1, 2 and 3*, because these perspectives are heavily linked to one another. So, the full expressive power of each perspective can only be achieved by considering its relations to the other perspectives. In this section, we will start from the metamodel of the functional and control-flow perspectives (Fig. 2.2) and step-by-step define the links with the data (Fig. 2.4) and resource (Fig. 2.6) perspectives. These links will open the door to expand the expressive power of the latter two perspectives even further. At the end, everything is integrated into one consistent metamodel that defines the new declarative process modeling language for loosely framed KiPs.

2.6.1   Integrating the Data Perspective

The rule patterns proposed by Caron et al. [67], which were already used in Sects. 2.5.3 and 2.5.4, also include two rule patterns (*D1* and *D2* in Table 2.5) that deal directly with the link between the data perspective (Fig. 2.4) the one hand and the functional/control-flow perspectives (Fig. 2.2) on the other hand. Yet, similar data patterns can be defined by taking inspiration from database applications, which are typically used to store and access the data in practical applications. Database query languages, like the popular Structured Query Language (SQL) [85], have defined a set of operations that can be performed on data: INSERT, SELECT, UPDATE and DELETE. This corresponds to how data records and their data attributes can be

Table 2.5 Six data patterns for KiPs

	Data pattern	Example
D1	Data-driven existence	If the patient has an open, displaced or unstable fracture, surgery will be performed at least once
D2	Data-driven relationships	If the patient is a minor, then consent is required from the legal guardian before surgery can be performed
D3	Insert data	If the patient does not have a patient file yet for this hospital, a new one needs to be created during the registration of a patient
D4	Read data	The doctor will need to examine the patient file during a consultation
D5	Update data	If the patient reports information that does not correspond to his/her patient file (e.g., a different allergy) when taking his/her medical history, the patient file will be updated
D6	Delete data	If a previously place internal fixation has been removed from the patient's arm, the data attribute in the patient's file stating that he/she has an internal fixation will be deleted

created, read, modified and removed during the execution of activities of a process. Based on these data operations from SQL, four additional data patterns have been formulated (*D3*, *D4*, *D5* and *D6* in Table 2.5).

Data patterns *D1* and *D2* essentially require the option for all constraint templates supported by the functional and control-flow perspectives to link them with data. As a result, constraints would not need to apply for all process executions, as is customary in most declarative languages, but can apply for a mere subset of executions. For example, the two examples from Table 2.5 can be modeled as *if('Open fracture = true' or 'Displaced fracture = true' or 'Unstable fracture = true') then AtLeast([Perform surgery], 1, 0, ∞)* and *if('Patient is a minor = true') then Precedence([Get consent from legal guardian], [Perform surgery], 0, ∞)*. To express that a constraint does apply to all process executions, it just needs to be linked with a trivial activation decision (i.e., always true). This will be represented in DeciClare by a constraint without the 'if'-part. For the constraint templates with a condition side (sometimes referred to as the source side), the activation decision on its own is not enough to activate the constraint (e.g., RespondedExistence, Response, Precedence…). Only the fulfilment of both the activation decision and condition of the constraint are enough for an activation. For example, consider a response constraint stating that if the patient has a displaced fracture, then surgery needs to be followed by applying a cast to the leg (i.e., *if('Displaced fracture = true') then Response([Perform surgery], [Apply cast], 0, ∞)*). For an activation of this constraint, the patient needs to have a displaced fracture *and* the doctors must have performed surgery. If one of these two conditions is not met, the constraint cannot be activated. An inactive constraint holds trivially (i.e., cannot be violated) and is commonly referred to as a vacuous satisfaction [26]. Hence, if the patient does not have a displaced fracture, the previous example constraint is not active and therefore vacuously satisfied.

Linking the functional, control-flow and data perspectives this way means that a constraint is always connected to an activation decision and the outcome of the decision is the activation of the constraint itself, while in the process making the LiteralExpression concept obsolete. This approach combines the power of the decision conditions to specify complex decisions based on data with the expressive power of the supported functional and control-flow perspectives as outcomes. This solution is similar to the decision-dependent constraints from Mertens et al. [55] and the first-order logic expressions from Maggi et al. [75], albeit here at a more general level. The decision-dependent constraints and first-order logic expressions can be seen as instantiations of the UnaryTest concept from Fig. 2.4. Linking the perspectives this way, has some consequences that need to be discussed in more detail and that sometimes also influence the design decisions made in previous section.

First, an important question that arises: does a constraint that is activated after some activities have been performed cover only the activities after its activation, or also the activities that preceded its activation? The latter interpretation, that constraints apply retroactively, might be useful when the models are used for conformance checking of past execution, but can make enforcing them practically impossible when using the model to execute the process. For example, a constraint stating that a certain activity can only be executed once, can be activated after it has already been executed multiple times. Requiring the executing process instances to satisfy constraints up to and after the constraint activation seriously limits the expressive power and does not correspond to how decisions are taken in real life processes. So, the applicability of an activated constraint will be defined as only the activities after the constraint activation.

A change to the definitions of the timed existence constraint templates is now required to maintain the consistency, because these templates specify that the time parameters (e.g., a and b) are relative to the process instance start, and thus, could have a retroactive effect. In order to prevent this, these parameters will be defined as relative to point in time when the constraint is activated. So for example, a timed 'AtLeast'-constraint could specify that a clinical examination must take place within the first hour after the patient was marked as 'yellow' during the triage (i.e., *if('Triage color = yellow') then AtLeast([Clinical examination of patient], 1, 0, 1 h)*), independent of the fact that the patient might have arrived 20 min before he/she was triaged. The parameters can still express time relative to the process instance start by having a trivial activation decision or an activation decision that evaluates as true at the start of the targeted process instances.

Second, having a decision to activate a constraint is one thing, but in some cases, it can be necessary to deactivate an activated constraint later on. Consider for example a constraint expressing that patients with a certain type of cancer need to receive at least six chemotherapy treatments. There are situations in which this constraint needs to be deactivated: if the patient reconsiders his consent after less than six treatments, if the patient experiences one or more complications after a couple of treatments and even the worst-case scenario when the patient deceases before at least six treatments have been administered. As these reasons could not be foreseen when formulating the activation decision for the constraint, a way to deactivate constraints is needed. So, every constraint will be given both an activation and deactivation decision. Of course, it is again allowed to be a trivial decision (i.e., always false) to represent a constraint that can never be deactivated. A constraint is not allowed to be violated as long it is activated but does not always need to be fulfilled completely like as illustrated in the following example. Suppose the patient wants to stop the treatment after just two of the six treatments, then the constraint is deactivated even though the minimum of six treatments prescribed by the constraint was never satisfied. Of course, if an activated constraint would put a maximum on the number of treatments, this maximum is not allowed to be broken in the timeframe between the activation and deactivation of the constraint, although it is allowed after the deactivation. A consequence of having both an activation and deactivation decision is that is possible that a constraint is activated and deactivated multiple times during one process instance. For example, take a constraint expressing that if a patient has fluid in his/her longs, then this needs to be drained within 3 min unless the fluid has already been drained or dissolved by itself (i.e., *if('Fluid in longs = true') then AtLeast([Drain fluid], 1, 0, 3 min) unless if('Fluid in longs = false'))*. Fluid is found the first time, the constraint is activated and the fluid will be drained. Afterwards, the constraint will be deactivated as the fluid has been drained. However, suppose the fluid immediately comes back. This activates the constraint again, leading to another deactivation after a second drainage.

Finally, a last unaddressed issue concerns the overlap in expressive power between the functional/control-flow and data perspectives (see requirement 4 in Sect. 2.4). The main reason for this overlap is that the decisions can specify the same conditions as the conditions of the relation templates. For example, consider the response constraint stating that taking an X-ray must be followed by a consultation (i.e., *Response([Take X-ray], [Doctor consultation], 0, ∞))*. This can also be expressed with an existence one constraint combined with an activation decision depending on the execution of the 'Take X-ray' activity (i.e., *if('Take X-ray has been executed = true') then AtLeast([Doctor consultation], 1), 0, ∞))*. This issue is resolved by not allowing decisions to use statements about the execution of events and activities. This eliminates the overlap, but at the same time reduces the expressive power of the resulting language. For instance, modeling a constraint like 'if surgery has been executed, then taking an X-ray will have to be executed at least 2 times' is no longer possible. To circumvent this side effect of the proposed solution, we will modify the relation templates to make such constraints possible once again. It comes down to allowing the relationship ends to be expressed in terms of existence templates. More specifically, the changes to the relation templates entail using branched existence (AtLeast), absence (AtMost), choice (AtLeastChoice) and AtMostChoice (see Sect. 2.6.3) templates to express both the condition and consequence sides. Like the branching principle discussed earlier, a logic expression connecting these templates with the logical conjunction and inclusive disjunction operations will be used as condition or consequence side. The previous example can now be modeled as follows: *Response(AtLeast([Perform surgery], 1), AtLeast([Take X-ray], 2), 0, ∞)*. As a side effect, the negative versions of the relation templates are no longer needed explicitly, since they can be expressed by using the normal templates with an absence 0 (AtMost 0) constraint as its consequence side. For example, consider a constraint stating that if an MRI has been taken, an X-ray cannot be taken afterwards. In Declare this would be written as *NotResponse([Take MRI], [Take X- ray])*, but we could now write this using the normal response-template as *Response(AtLeast([Take MRI], 1), AtMost([Take X- ray], 0), 0, ∞)*. The end result of this set of changes to the relation templates can express everything we could before the changes but has eliminated the overlap and adds even more expressive power by making it possible to express relations between multiple executions of events.

Now that support for the first two data patterns has been added, the last four patterns (*D3, D4, D5* and *D6*) need to be addressed. For each of these data patterns two constraint templates can be defined to express whether this operation must occur or cannot occur. This results in the following constraint templates: RequiredInsertion/ProhibitedInsertion, RequiredRead/ProhibitedRead, RequiredUpdate/ProhibitedUpdate and RequiredDeletion/ProhibitedDeletion. The templates relate data structures to activities of the process. The parameters of these templates are branched in a similar manner as for the control-flow constraint templates: a logical expression using activities (inclusive disjunction) and a logical expression of data structures (inclusive disjunction). Additionally, each of these templates has time parameters and an activation and deactivation decision. The last four examples of Table 2.5 can now be modeled as follows:

- D3: *if('Patient has been to this hospital before = false') then RequiredInsertion([Register patient], [Patient file], 0, ∞)*
- D4: *RequiredRead([Doctor consultation], [Patient file], 0, ∞)*
- D5: *optional RequiredUpdate([Take medical history of patient], [Patient file], 0, ∞)*
- D6: *RequiredDeletion([Remove fixation], [Patient file/fixations], 0, ∞)*

2.6.2 Integrating the Resource Perspective

The resource patterns defined by [10, 80, 81] were used in Sect. 2.5.6 to define a resource perspective for DeciClare. However, several patterns could not yet be discussed as they require links to the other perspectives. Table 2.6 presents the remaining resource patterns relevant to loosely framed and KiPs. Again, an additional resource pattern was added (denoted by an asterisk). This pattern is a variation on the existing authorization pattern. The original pattern covers the authorization of a role to execute a certain task, while the added authorization pattern covers the authorization of roles to take certain decisions. As KiPs typically involve multiple process workers, establishing these authorization rules can be crucial in order to successfully execute the process.

The metamodel of the ConDec-R language (Fig. 2.5) directly satisfies resource pattern *R5*, so a similar solution will now be added to the metamodel of the resource perspective of DeciClare (Fig. 2.6). Analogous to how support was added to express resource availabilities, new constraint templates are added that use branching and upper/lower bounds to express resource allocations: *AtLeastUsage* and *AtMostUsage*.

Table 2.6 Six additional resource patterns linking the resource perspective to the other perspectives

	Resource pattern	Example
R4	Direct allocation	Brain surgery is performed in operation room no.1
R5	Role-based allocation	Applying a cast requires at least one doctor or one nurse
R6	Activity-based authorization	A surgeon is authorized to perform surgery
R7	Decision-based authorization*	A doctor is authorized to decide whether or not surgery to be performed
R8	Automatic execution (no human resources)	Monitoring the heartrate of the patient is executed by the heartrate monitor machine
R9	Separation of duties	For surgery, one person cannot take on both the surgeon and anesthesiologist roles

They have five parameters: a logical expression using activities (inclusive disjunction), a logical expression using resources (inclusive disjunction), a lower or upper bound, and two time parameters. They can express that a certain activity needs at least or at most a certain number of resources (possibly, but not necessarily, of the same type). For example, it can state that applying a cast requires at least one doctor or one nurse: *AtLeastUsage([Apply cast], [Doctor or Nurse], 1, 0, ∞)*.

No further changes are required to support the direct allocation of resources (*R4*), as this is done analogous to the direct availability of resources (*R1*). For example, stating that all brain surgeries must be performed in operating room no.1 can be expressed as *AtLeastUsage([Perform brain surgery], ["operating room no. 1"], 1, 0, ∞)*.

The authorization patterns (e.g., *R6*, *R7* and *R8*) are also not yet supported by the metamodel. To implement these patterns two additional pairs of constraint templates are added: *(Not)DecisionAuthorization* and *(Not)ActivityAuthorization*. These templates have as input on the one hand a logical expression using resources (inclusive disjunction) and on the other hand, respectively, a constraint or an activity. They express that the connected resources have authorization to take the decision connected to a certain constraint or execute a certain activity. The examples for *R6*, *R7* and *R8* from Table 2.6 can now be modeled as follows: *ActivityAuthorization([Orthopedic surgeon], [Perform surgery])), DecisionAuthorization([Doctor], [if('Displaced fracture? = true' or 'Open fracture? = true') then AtLeast([Perform surgery], 1, 0, ∞)]))* and *ActivityAuthorization([Heart rate monitor], [Monitor heart rate]))*. The last template can also be used to, for example, express that an expert system has authorization to diagnose a patient autonomously (i.e., *ActivityAuthorization([Expert system], [Diagnose patient])).*

The final resource pattern is the one that expresses the principle of separation of duties (*R9*). To support this pattern, two more resource constraint templates are introduced. The *ResourceEquality* and *ResourceInequality* constraint templates are connected to two or more pairs of logical expressions, each consisting of one resource expression (inclusive disjunction) and one activity expression (inclusive

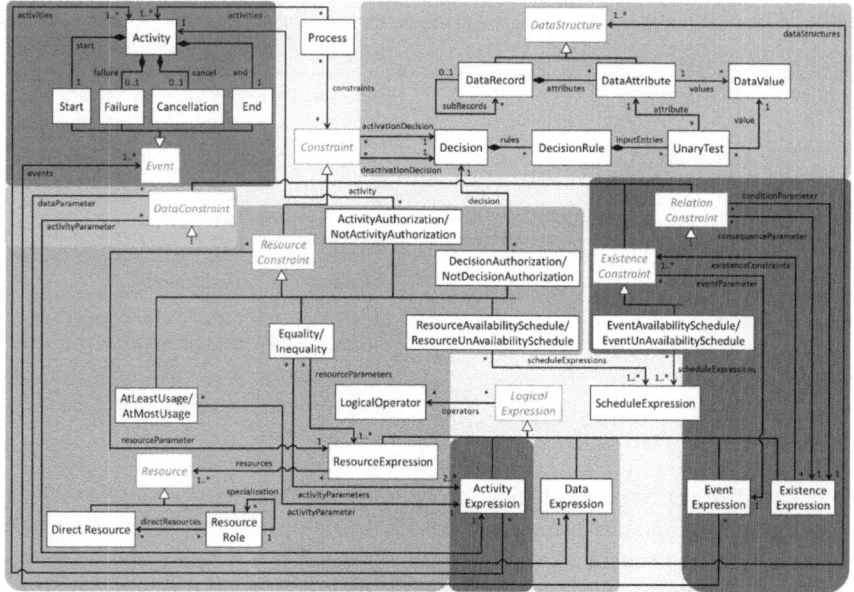

Fig. 2.7 The metamodel of the DeciClare language (blue = functional, purple = control-flow, orange = data and green = resource)

disjunction). This allows for expressing that resources from certain activities must be the same or must be different, respectively, as the resources in some other activities. Consider the example from Table 2.6 for *R9*, this can now be modeled as *ResourceInequality([Orthopedic surgeon or Anesthesiologist], [Perform surgery])*. An example of a resource equality on the other hand, would be to express that the surgeon that performed the surgery needs to be the same doctor as the one that does the follow-up examination of the patient (i.e., *ResourceEquality([Orthopedic surgeon], [Perform surgery or Doctor consultation])*).

2.6.3   DeciClare

The metamodel of the DeciClare modeling language, which fully integrates the functional/control-flow, data and resource perspectives presented earlier, is presented in Fig. 2.7. Some constraint templates without additional relations have been omitted to improve readability. An Ecore implementation of the complete metamodel has been made available[3].

As summary of the solutions for each of the perspectives, the resulting constraint templates are presented in Table 2.7, Table 2.8 and Table 2.9. For Table 2.7, the second

---

[3]DeciClare_ecore.zip available at https://doi.org/10.1016/j.eswa.2017.06.024

column contains the constraint templates from the most expressive Declare extension Declare^{++}. In Table 2.8 and Table 2.9 this column was omitted, as both perspectives are not supported by Declare^{++}. The last column of each table relates the constraint template to the corresponding patterns from Table 2.2, Table 2.3, Table 2.4, Table 2.5 and Table 2.6. The parameters X, I, C and B define the logical operators that can be used in the parameter expressions of the template as a result of the branching concept. The used letter refers to the option to use the exclusive disjunction (X), inclusive disjunction (I), conjunction (C) or both the inclusive disjunction and conjunction (B). The numerical bound enforced by some templates is expressed by the parameter n. The time interval linked to the Timed Declare definitions is represented by parameters a and b. The set of schedule expressions is denoted by S (*T6*). To save space, the activation and deactivation decisions for each constraint template and their optional versions have been omitted. The optional versions of each of the templates (rule pattern *G*) are of course still supported in the same way as the respective mandatory versions. In addition to presenting the solutions for the functional and control-flow perspectives of DeciClare, Table 2.7 also shows the results of a systematic review based on the principle of domain appropriateness (i.e., *requirement 4*) of the existing constraint templates. Some of the templates from Declare have been renamed in order to clarify their meaning and to emphasize the symmetry of the templates, while others have been omitted because they are either redundant (i.e., exclusive allowance) or syntactic sugar. The latter means that they can be easily expressed in terms of the other templates. Syntactic sugar can be categorized as construct redundancy, and thus, needs to be avoided in order to meet *requirement 4*. It is something that could be reintroduced when defining a concrete syntax to improve usability, but it does not belong in the metamodel of the language.

Table 2.7 The control-flow constraint templates of Declare ++ and DeciClare

Type	Declare^{++}	DeciClare	Patterns
Existence templates	existence(n, Activity, a, b)	AtLeast(I, n, a, b)	*A, E, T1*
	absence(n, Activity, a, b)	AtMost(B, n, a, b)	*A, E, T1*
	exactly(n, Activity, a, b)	*(removed: syntactic sugar)*	–
	init(Activity)	*(removed: syntactic sugar)*	–
	last(Activity)	*(removed: syntactic sugar)*	–
	choice(n, I, a, b)	AtLeastChoice(B, n, a, b)	*B, T1*
	exclusive choice(n, I, a, b)	*(removed: syntactic sugar due inclusion of AtMostChoice)*	–
	–	AtMostChoice(B, n, a, b)	*B, T1*
	–	EventAvailabilitySchedule(I, S)	*E, T6*
	–	EventUnavailabilitySchedule(I, S)	*E, T6*

(continued)

Table 2.7 (continued)

Type	Declare++	DeciClare	Patterns
Relation templates	responded existence(I_1, I_2)	RespondedPresence(B_1, B_2)	*B, D, E*
	responded absence(I_1, I_2)	*(removed: expressed as RespondedPresence with AtMost-consequence)*	–
	coexistence(I_1, I_2, a, b)	*(removed: syntactic sugar)*	–
	not coexistence(I_1, I_2, a, b)	*(removed: syntactic sugar)*	–
	response(I_1, I_2, a, b)	Response(B_1, B_2, a, b)	*C, D, E, T2*
	not response(I_1, I_2, a, b)	*(removed: expressed as Response with AtMost-consequence)*	–
	chain response(I_1, I_2, a, b)	ChainResponse(B_1, B_2, a, b)	*C, D, E, T2*
	not chain response(I_1, I_2, a, b)	*(removed: expressed as ChainResponse with AtMost-consequence)*	–
	alternate response(I_1, I_2, a, b)	AlternateResponse(B_1, B_2, a, b)	*C, E, T2*
	precedence(I_1, I_2, a, b)	Precedence(B_1, B_2, a, b)	*C, D, E, T2*
	not precedence(I_1, I_2, a, b)	*(removed: expressed as Precedence with AtMost-consequence)*	–
	chain precedence(I_1, I_2, a, b)	ChainPrecedence(B_1, B_2, a, b)	*C, D, E, T2*
	not chain precedence(I_1, I_2, a, b)	*(removed: expressed as ChainPrecedence with AtMost-consequence)*	–
	alternate precedence(I_1, I_2, a, b)	AlternatePrecedence(B_1, B_2, a, b)	*C, E, T2*
	succession(I_1, I_2, a, b)	*(removed: syntactic sugar)*	–
	not succession(I_1, I_2, a, b)	*(removed: syntactic sugar)*	–
	chain succession(I_1, I_2, a, b)	*(removed: syntactic sugar)*	–
	not chain succession(I_1, I_2, a, b)	*(removed: syntactic sugar)*	–
	alternate succession(I_1, I_2, a, b)	*(removed: syntactic sugar)*	–
	–	AtLeastLag(B_1, B_2, n)	*E, T2/3/4/5/7*
	–	AtMostLag(B_1, B_2, n)	*E, T2/3/4/5/7*

Table 2.8 The data perspective constraint templates of DeciClare

Type	DeciClare	Patterns
Data templates	RequiredInsertion(I_{act}, I_{data}, a, b)	*D3*
	ProhibitedInsertion(I_{act}, I_{data}, a, b)	*D3*
	RequiredRead(I_{act}, I_{data}, a, b)	*D4*
	ProhibitedRead(I_{act}, I_{data}, a, b)	*D4*
	RequiredUpdate(I_{act}, I_{data}, a, b)	*D5*
	ProhibitedUpdate(I_{act}, I_{data}, a, b)	*D5*
	RequiredDeletion(I_{act}, I_{data}, a, b)	*D6*
	ProhibitedDeletion(I_{act}, I_{data}, a, b)	*D6*

Table 2.9 The resource perspective constraint templates of DeciClare

Type	DeciClare	Patterns
Resource templates	AtLeastAvailable(I_{res}, n, a, b)	*R1, R2*
	AtMostAvailable(I_{res}, n, a, b)	*R1, R2*
	ResourceAvailabilitySchedule(I_{res}, S)	*T6*
	ResourceUnavailabilitySchedule(I_{res}, S)	*T6*
	SimultaneousCapacity(res, n)	*R3*
	AtLeastUsage(A, I_{res}, n, a, b)	*R4, R5*
	AtMostUsage(A, I_{res}, n, a, b)	*R4, R5*
	ActivityAuthorization(I_{res}, act)	*R6, R8*
	NoActivityAuthorization(I_{res}, act)	*R6, R8*
	DecisionAuthorization(I_{res}, constraint)	*R7, R8*
	NoDecisionAuthorization(I_{res}, constraint)	*R7, R8*
	ResourceEquality($[I_{res}, I_{act}]_{2..}*$)	*R9*
	ResourceInequality($[I_{res}, I_{act}]_{2..}*$)	*R9*

2.7   Evaluation

Hevner et al. [38] and Peffers et al. [86] present several types of evaluation that can be used to evaluate design science artifacts. A combination of expert evaluation and an illustrative scenario Peffers et al. has been used to evaluate the artifact of this chapter, which is the abstract syntax of the DeciClare modeling language. More specifically, domain experts have evaluated the abstract syntax with the help of the realistic arm fracture case, presented in Sect. 2.5.1, as application scenario. The goal of this evaluation was to validate the effectiveness of the abstract syntax of the DeciClare language. The reasons for including certain modeling concepts in the abstract syntax have already been discussed in Sects. 2.4–2.6 and were each based on either literature or practical examples (i.e., informed arguments [38]). In the first subsection, the set-up of the evaluation will be discussed. In the subsequent subsections the results of the evaluation concerning different quality types will be presented.

2.7.1   The Evaluation Set-up

The effectiveness of the design artifact, the metamodel of the DeciClare modeling language, can be assessed by applying the Conceptual Modeling Quality Framework (CMQF) [54]. This framework proposes several quality types based on what are called the quality cornerstones of conceptual modeling. The cornerstone that serves as the subject of our evaluation is the DeciClare metamodel, which in terms of the CMQF corresponds to a physical language that attempts to allow users to create a faithful representation of relevant concepts and phenomena in the physical domain, in this case loosely framed and KiPs.

In order to evaluate the DeciClare metamodel both directly and indirectly a realistic healthcare process of diagnosing and treating patients with suspected arm fractures was introduced. Because a concrete syntax of DeciClare was not yet available, the textual representations of the proposed metamodel, as used throughout this chapter, were used to serve as a temporary implementation of a concrete syntax for the DeciClare language. To make it as easy as possible for the participants, the metamodel instantiations were subsequently translated to more understandable natural language (see Appendix B for the original DeciClare model). For example, the constraint stating that surgery must be performed within 1 h if the symptoms for acute compartment syndrome have been fulfilled was originally modeled as "*AtLeast(Perform surgery, 1, 0, 1 h) activateIf[[Has acute compartment syndrome? = true]] deactivateIf[False]*" and now becomes "*If('Has acute compartment syndrome? = true') then Perform surgery must be performed at least 1 time within at most 1 h*". The original model of the case was based on the available literature and contained 15 activities, 11 resources, 15 data attributes and 79 constraints (35 functional/control-flow, 37 resource, 7 data and no guideline constraints) using 10 different constraint templates of the 22 available across all perspectives (not counting the mandatory/optional, positive/negative and at most/at least versions separately).

Using both the metamodel and the instantiation of the model, the CMQF framework can be used to evaluate the effectiveness of the language with three different quality types: perceived semantic quality, pragmatic quality and language-domain appropriateness. The perceived semantic quality of the case model represents the extent to which the model accurately and completely captures the domain knowledge of the experts, within the scope of the modeling task at hand [87]. During the interviews issues with the semantic quality of the case model were treated as opportunities. They allow for discussions on the exact origin of the encountered issues and possible solutions. For instance, problems with the completeness of the language could be revealed, if it is not possible to formulate a satisfactory solution (i.e., missing concepts or relations in the DeciClare metamodel). The pragmatic quality on the other hand captures the extent to which the experts completely and accurately understand the parts of the case model that are relevant to their roles in the actual process. Basically, this gives an idea of the usefulness and value of the case model to the stakeholders of the process, and per extension of modeling with DeciClare in general.

Both perceived semantic quality and pragmatic quality indirectly evaluate the DeciClare metamodel by means of the developed model. The language-domain appropriateness quality type of the CMQF has as object of interest the metamodel of the language. It is the quality type related to the relationship between the physical language and the physical domain. However, an objective measurement of this relationship is impossible, because the universe of discourse related to the domain of loosely framed and KiPs is impossible to capture in its entirety. To circumvent this issue, a more subjective quality type can be used as approximation: the perceived language-domain appropriateness [54]. This quality type states that the metamodel, as understood by the users/modelers, must be appropriate to the understanding of the real-world universe of discourse by these users/modelers and for the ultimate use of the models created with the modeling language. This can be assessed by domain experts, who possess the in-depth knowledge of loosely framed KiPs to assess the appropriateness of the DeciClare metamodel to allow creating faithful representations of such processes.

By way of several semi-structured interviews with domain experts, all three quality types were evaluated for the DeciClare modeling language (see Appendix C for the interview protocol). In the first part of the interview, the expert was introduced to the research project and the DeciClare modeling language. In the second part, a brief introduction to the arm fracture case and its scope was given, followed by some time to thoroughly read the case description. When the experts were fully aware of the scope of the case and sufficiently understood the modeling language, they were presented with the natural language model of the case. All the rules of the model were discussed one by one as part of the semantic quality evaluation. If a rule did not conform to reality, corrections were discussed. In the last part of the interview the pragmatic quality of the model was discussed followed by a general discussion about the perceived language-domain appropriateness of the modeling language. The arm fracture case takes place in the emergency and orthopedic departments of hospitals. Therefore, four medical professionals that fulfill different roles along these departments in three of the biggest hospitals in Ghent were interviewed as domain experts: a surgeon from the AZ Sint-Lucas hospital, an emergency nurse/process quality promotor from the Ghent University Hospital and both an orthopedic surgeon and an orthopedic surgeon in training (intern) from the AZ Maria Middelares hospital in Ghent. The first three were very experienced and offered detailed insight into the process in practice, while the orthopedic surgeon in training was able to cast a different light on the process based on his training and his recent emergence into the complexity of real-life cases.

2.7.2   *Evaluating the Perceived Semantic Quality*

In order to verify the sematic quality of the model the participants were instructed to validate the constraints of the model in a per-context (e.g., all relevant constraints when a patient with a finger fracture enters the emergency department) way on their correctness and completeness. This revealed some interesting feedback on the model of the case: new activities (e.g., 'Prescribe stomach protecting drug'), data values (e.g., 'Displaced fracture') and constraints were added, while others were modified and some even removed. The reasons ranged from a lack of detail in the original model concerning certain treatments and decisions to a sense that certain deadlines were difficult to enforce or merely hospital policies that differ from hospital to hospital. All of the suggested changes could be incorporated into the model with the available modeling constructs supplied by the DeciClare metamodel as to the eventual satisfaction of the experts. So, this did not expose any issues concerning the completeness of the language. After each interview the model was updated with additional insights, resulting in a final model containing 25 activities, 17 resources, 21 data attributes and 282 constraints (126 functional/control-flow, 115 resource, 7 data and 34 guideline constraints) using 16 different constraint templates (see Appendix D). Most of the DeciClare examples used throughout this were taken from this updated model of the arms fracture case.

2.7.3   *Evaluating the Pragmatic Quality*

The pragmatic quality of the case model assesses the extent to which the experts understood the model and were able to use it. To this purpose, the experts were asked to identify examples of conforming and non-conforming process instances based on the model. All of them were able to perform this task satisfactory. For the non-conforming examples, they were also able to pinpoint the violated constraint or set of constraints.

Furthermore, the experts were asked if they could use the model to support their daily job. The responses confirmed the usefulness of the model. They all agree with the statement made earlier in this chapter, that it can be a valuable tool when training new personnel. The orthopedic surgeon in training also added that he had not encountered anything similar during his education and training. They were taught using all sorts of specific clinical pathways [88], but never got a higher level view of the process. He agreed that a model like this could have the potential to significantly shorten the internship duration, as they would no longer be limited to gaining experience from shadowing cases of more experienced doctors. Also, the experts see it as a great way to communicate changes to the process, be it due to policy changes, new diagnostic tests or new treatments. However, it was noted that the direct value of the model for a certain process actor somewhat diminishes as the experience level of the process actor rises. This was to be expected, as a rising experience level means that the knowledge made explicit by the model becomes more and more known. So less experienced process actors will be able to learn more from the model, than those with more experience. Yet, as noted by the emergency nurse, more experienced process actors can still get more insight into how other process actors, fulfilling different roles, make decisions. Her role in the process is to prepare the patient before seeing the doctor and provide support throughout. The model could help her identify and acquire the specific bits of information that the doctors will need in subsequent activities faster.

The experts were also asked how they currently use the information described in the model in their daily job. While they acknowledged the tacit nature of the knowledge by referring to its application as a sort of autopilot mode, they did say that they think more in terms of clinical pathways due to the nature of their training. The constraints expressed by the model refer to one or a few activities directly or to a relation between them, however, the experts would group them more according to certain clinical pathways (e.g., a Colles' fracture). An interesting feature to consider would be to allow filters on the model, showing only the constraints that apply for specified data values. This would allow the constraints for each clinical pathway to be presented separately, while still being able to connect them to the complete process. This is somewhat similar to how Maggi et al. [89] filtered their Declare models based on previously executed activities to make them more understandable. Additionally, they indicated that in reality many decisions also come down to patient preferences. Typically, the patient is directly or indirectly responsible for much of the variability present in a healthcare process. For example, the constraints in the model do not account for patients that refuse treatment. Of course, the patient preferences can be represented by data values, but this would make the decision logic of the affected constraints more complex. The experts agreed that for communication purposes this would be unfavorable, but for analysis and training purposes it could be very useful to know exactly which decisions need to account for patient preference and which do not.

2.7.4 Evaluating the Language-Domain Appropriateness

In the last part of the interview, the DeciClare metamodel textual representations were discussed independently of the presented case. The experts agreed that the language is sufficiently expressive to also model the real underlying process without the limitations put on the scope (i.e., the complete emergency services process). They feel that the model would become a lot more complex, but that the added complexity would be in proportion to the added complexity of the real-world process. When considering applying the technique to other healthcare processes that fit the mold of flexible and KiPs, they were unable to think of examples (i.e., processes or types of constraints) that could not be expressed using the DeciClare language. The lack of identified construct deficits [58] at this point or during the discussion of the case model, allows us to conclude that there are no apparent issues with the completeness of the language. Also, no construct excesses [58] were uncovered, since real-life examples of each of the constraint templates could be given. Of course, this is because special attention was given to these properties during the design of the language.

One expert did, however, mention that after discussing some of the modeling elements from Declare that were left out due to being syntactic sugar, she would prefer to have these elements included to simplify the models. The example that we discussed was to include the 'Init' template, from the Declare language, to express that the patient registration must happen as the first activity of a process instance (*Init([Register patient])*). Instead, this was expressed by 24 precedence relations between the patient registration activity and every other activity (i.e., *Precedence([AtLeast([Register patient], 1)], [AtLeast([Take medical history of patient], 1)], 0, ∞)* and the same for the 23 other activities). As stated in Sect. 2.6.3, we are certainly open to adding these types of modeling elements as part of the eventual concrete syntax of the language. Introducing the Init/Last templates and the 'exactly' versions of each of the AtLeast/AtMost templates would have reduced the final case model from 282 to 218 constraints (78 functional/control-flow, 99 resource and 7 data and 34 guideline constraints). However, these templates were not included in the temporary concrete syntax used for the purpose of this evaluation, because it was a direct instantiation of the metamodel of DeciClare.

When considering the DeciClare language as a whole, the experts were most intrigued by how the different perspectives complemented each other. A good example of this from the case model were the rules that modeled what should happen when a patient has a confirmed displaced wrist or forearm fracture. The normal treatment involves surgery to reposition the broken bone (i.e., *if('Displaced fracture = true' or 'Open fracture = true') then AtLeast([Perform surgery], 1, 0, ∞)*), which requires at least a free operating room (i.e., *AtLeastUsage([Perform surgery], [operating room], 1)*), a surgeon (i.e., *AtLeastUsage([Perform surgery], [orthopedic surgeon], 1)*), an anesthesiologist (i.e., *AtLeastUsage([Perform surgery], [anesthesiologist], 1)*) and a surgical assistant or one or more OR or scrub nurses (i.e., *AtLeastUsage([Perform surgery], [surgical assistant or scrub nurse], 1)* and *AtLeastUsage([Perform surgery], [OR nurse], 1)*). But we also modeled the frequently occurring situation where the operating time (i.e., the time for which all the necessary resources need to be available) is not yet available (i.e., *if['Displaced fracture? = true' and 'Operating time available? = false' and 'Confirmed Fracture? = Wrist'] or ['Displaced fracture = true' and 'Operating time available = false' and 'Confirmed Fracture = Forearm']) then Precedence([[AtLeast([Apply cast], 1) or AtLeast([Apply splint], 1)] and AtLeast([Stay in patient room], 1)], [AtLeast([Perform surgery], 1)], 0, ∞) unless if('Operating time available = true')*). Instead, the responsible doctor will order a temporary cast or splint to be applied (by himself or a nurse) to bridge the time until the operating time becomes available again. This situation could be modeled completely in DeciClare, because it supports and combines the necessary decisions, functional/control-flow restrictions and resource reasoning to express it. Therefore, the general conclusion of the experts was that the perceived model-domain appropriateness of DeciClare is satisfactory and that it is sufficiently expressive to model loosely framed and KiPs with the needed level of detail.

2.8 Positioning of DeciClare in the Research Domain

A summary of the expressive power of all languages and extensions used in this chapter in relation to the requirements of Sect. 2.4 and their operationalization by means of patterns in Sects. 2.5 and 2.6 is presented in Table 2.10. When a pattern is covered by the language this is denoted by '+', when unaddressed by '-' and when not applicable by '/'. In some cases, a certain pattern is somewhat addressed, but not to the full extent, which is denoted by '±'.

The language proposed in this work, DeciClare, can be classified as a *mixed-perspective* process modeling language, as opposed to a *multi-perspective* process modeling language. The former combines perspectives by integrating the metamodels of the perspectives into one resulting metamodel. The latter combines perspectives by using them side by side, keeping the metamodels of these languages separated. Coloured Petri nets [90] is another example of a mixed-perspective language, as it uses one integrated metamodel to combine the control-flow perspective of regular Petri nets with a data perspective. The pockets of flexibility approaches of Sadiq et al. [91] and De Smedt et al. [92] are more examples of mixed-perspective approaches. The Declare extensions Declare^{++}, ConDec-R, data-aware Declare and Declare based on LTL-FO can also be classified as mixed-perspective modeling languages. The difference with DeciClare is that they cover at most three perspectives, where this work covers the main four. On the other hand, Maggi et al. [93] and Frank [94] are examples of multi-perspective approaches combining perspectives related to representation (also called representation paradigms). For Maggi et al., either an imperative or declarative representation is chosen, depending on the characteristics of each sub-process in isolation. The two are never combined into one model. In Frank, the metamodels of the different perspectives remain separated, with a meta-metamodel relating all the metamodels.

The DeciClare language does not fall into the category of hybrid languages. Within business process modeling research, the category of 'hybrid process modeling languages' is used to signify the combination of imperative and declarative modeling languages into one approach [16, 91–93, 95]. The idea is that some of the information can be better expressed using an imperative language, while for other parts this is true when using a declarative language. So, they combine two (or more) paradigms, in the form of either a multi- or mixed-perspective language, to *represent* the information contained by the model. DeciClare uses only one paradigm for representation, the declarative paradigm, but instead focuses on combining different *content* related perspectives (like Coloured Petri nets).

Table 2.10 A comparison of the languages used in this paper based on the requirements from Sect. 2.4 and their operationalization as patterns from Sect. 2.5 and 2.6

		Declare (Pesic 2008)	Timed Declare (Westergaard et al. 2012)	TBDeclare (Di Ciccio et al. 2016)	ConDec-R (Jiménez-Ramírez et al. 2013)	Data-aware Declare (Borrego et al. 2013)	Declare++ (Montali 2010; Montali et al. 2014)	Declare based on LTL-FO (Maggi et al. 2013)	DMN (Object Management Group 2013)	Declare-R-DMN (Mertens et al. 2016)	DeciClare
1	A	+	+	+	+	+	+	+	/	+	+
	B	+	+	+	+	+	+	+	/	+	+
	C	+	+	+	+	+	+	+	/	+	+
	D	+	+	+	+	+	+	+	/	+	+
	E	-	-	±	-	-	+	-	/	-	+
	F	-	-	-	-	-	-	-	/	-	+
	G	+	+	+	+	+	+	+	/	+	+
	T1	-	+	-	-	-	-	-	/	-	+
	T2	-	+	-	-	-	+	-	/	-	+
	T3	-	-	-	-	-	-	-	/	-	+
	T4	-	-	-	-	-	-	-	/	-	+
	T5	-	-	-	-	-	-	-	/	-	+
	T6	-	-	-	-	-	-	-	/	-	+
	T7	-	-	-	-	-	-	-	/	-	+
2		-	-	-	-	±	±	+	+	+	+
3	R1	-	-	-	-	-	-	-	/	-	+
	R2	-	-	-	+	-	-	-	/	+	+
	R3	-	-	-	-	-	-	-	/	-	+
4	R4	-	-	-	-	-	-	-	/	-	+
	R5	-	-	-	+	-	-	-	/	+	+
	R6	-	-	-	-	-	-	-	/	-	+
	R7	-	-	-	-	-	-	-	/	+	+
	R8	-	-	-	-	-	-	-	/	-	+
	R9	-	-	-	-	-	-	-	/	-	+
	D1	-	-	-	-	+	+	+	/	±	+
	D2	-	-	-	-	+	+	+	/	+	+
	D3	-	-	-	-	-	-	-	/	-	+
	D4	-	-	-	-	-	-	-	/	-	+
	D5	-	-	-	-	-	-	-	/	-	+
	D6	-	-	-	-	-	-	-	/	-	+

2.9 Conclusion

In this chapter the metamodel of the mixed-perspective declarative modeling language DeciClare has been presented. This metamodel is the final step in a journey that started with the formulation of requirements of a modeling language for loosely framed and KiPs. These requirements were translated into sets of smaller requirements (i.e., patterns) based on relevant literature, which represent the operationalization of the original requirements. Subsequently, the patterns were analyzed one by one and addressed. Although several existing languages already targeted this type of processes, none could offer the means to model all of its intricacies as specified by the requirements. The foundation for the DeciClare language was the popular declarative process modeling language Declare. Based on the requirements, an evaluation was performed to identify the aspects supported and unsupported by Declare. Because the Declare language received many standalone extensions since its conception, the relevant extensions were also evaluated in the same way. This helped reveal exactly those parts that could be reused and those that necessitated new solutions. After the development of separate solutions for the different perspectives in response to the requirements, an integration step was performed. The integration of the perspectives is an important step for the academic and practical applicability of declarative languages. The myriad of standalone extensions might each add support for some specific aspects, but an approach combining of all of these extensions is a vital step to capturing these processes completely in a process model.

An essential aspect of modeling KiPs is, of course, modeling the knowledge itself. This knowledge governs the process and all of its numerous variations. As it is typically of a tacit nature, it is paramount that a language to model these processes offers a way to explicitly represent the decision logic that expresses it. DeciClare links each declarative constraint with decision logic that can make the constraint active and that can deactivate an active constraint. Process models can therefore represent the process very precisely, as well as the knowledge governing it. This facilitates the sharing of knowledge with other knowledge workers and with other stakeholders of the process (e.g., the patient). Additionally, a more uniform and transparent service can be offered when the knowledge workers are more informed, and they have a way to communicate changes to the process at their disposal.

Along the way, this work also makes several contributions to the research domain in the form of other metamodels. The first metamodel that was presented is the one of the Declare language (Fig. 2.1). Although a partial metamodel for Declare had been proposed before [65], it was not fully compatible with the original definitions of the language and its corresponding modeling tool. This metamodel was subsequently enriched with additional concepts and relations in response to the requirements. The resulting model (Fig. 2.2) presents a direct extension of the Declare language, since it originally only covered the functional and control-flow perspectives. When considering the addition of a data perspective, the concepts from DMN and a simple data representation were used to create a metamodel for the data side (Fig. 2.4). And finally, a metamodel of the resource perspective was presented in Fig. 2.6. This model was based on the proposed metamodel of ConDec-R extension (Fig. 2.5) for Declare, for which a metamodel was also lacking in literature.

The effectiveness of the abstract syntax of the DeciClare language was evaluated by way of semi-structured interviews with domain experts. An example of a loosely framed and KiP was used (i.e., a simplification of the emergency services process only considering patients with possible fractures in the arms) to make the discussions and questions more relatable for the experts. Based on a general explanation of DeciClare, the case description and a textual DeciClare model of the case, the language-domain appropriateness of the language was assessed. The semantic and pragmatic quality of the case model were discussed, and afterwards a general discussion took place about the DeciClare language. This led to two main takeaways.

The first conclusion that can be drawn from the evaluation is that the DeciClare language appears to be sufficiently expressive to model loosely framed and KiPs. This will be further verified in the future by using DeciClare to model several more loosely framed KiPs (cf. chapter 4), preferably from different domains (e.g., legal profession). The original case model was enriched during each of the interviews, but nothing was encountered that could not be expressed in DeciClare. The domain experts saw no potential problems for the model of the case to be expanded to represent the unrestricted diagnosis and treatment process in the emergency service department, apart from the proportional increase in complexity. Additionally, they were unable to come up with constraints that could not be captured by a DeciClare model but might occur in different processes of this type.

The second conclusion is that the experts deemed modeling the processes with DeciClare useful for training and communication purposes. It can be a tool to make these processes, which are generally perceived as black boxes by management, more transparent to all stakeholders. It also allows for process actors to anticipate the needs of other process actors more correctly, because the models can offer insight into their role in the process and their corresponding needs. However, experience plays a vital role here. Inexperienced process actors will benefit more from the added insight, as more experienced actors already know much of the information relayed by the model.

In general, DeciClare offers modelers a new way to model loosely framed KiPs. Although it is a new language, it still has a familiar feel to it because existing modeling concepts were integrated whenever possible. Compared to alternative languages, the main advantage of DeciClare stems from its integration of the different perspectives of the process. Most of the languages targeting the same types of processes offer only one perspective to the process, resulting in important information getting lost during the modeling phase (as illustrated by Table 2.10). DeciClare allows each of the essential perspectives of the processes to be represented, as well as the links between these perspectives. This is somewhat similar to what the BPMN/DMN language extension attempts to do for tightly framed processes. BPMN/DMN also combines the functional, control-flow, resource and data perspectives, but using the imperative modeling paradigm. On the flipside, approaches like DeciClare and BPMN/DMN introduce a lot of added complexity. It is a typical tradeoff between simplicity and expressive power. In case of DeciClare, we feel that the latter is justified because the targeted processes are inherently complex. The resulting models are still an abstraction of reality that offers a view of the process with reduced complexity, but they are also comprehensive enough to represent the most important intricacies of the process. Additionally, we envision most practical applications of these models (e.g., process mining, simulation, conformance checking and run-time support) to be supported by way of (semi-)automated techniques.

Finally, the DeciClare language was positioned in the business process modeling domain using several possible classifications. The first classification is according to the types of processes that the language targets, in this cases loosely framed KiPs. Of course, this was a design decision. The second classification positions the language according to what type of perspectives are combined in the language and how these different perspectives are combined. DeciClare can be classified as a *mixed-perspective* modeling language, because multiple *content* perspectives (i.e., functional, control-flow, data and resource) are integrated into one metamodel. The last classification is according to the usage scenarios supported by the language. At design-time it provides the means to convert tacit knowledge generally associated with loosely framed processes to explicit knowledge, allowing this knowledge encapsulated in the models to be communicated with others. The language makes it possible to explain and justify why things are done a certain way, by making the decision logic transparent for all stakeholders. In an execution context it facilitates conformance checking of past and present process executions.

2.10 Limitations and Future Work

Firstly, the scope of this work was limited to the abstract syntax of the modeling language. A visual syntax for a modeling language requires a different research approach (i.e., cognitive instead of semantic) and a different evaluation, and so we chose to split the two into separate research steps that each can be performed in greater depth. Therefore, the next step in this research cycle will be to develop a visual syntax for the DeciClare language.

A second limitation is intrinsic to declarative modeling, namely that the models tend to be complex and difficult to understand for human users. Of course, the choice for a good visual syntax will also play a role in this, but an extended metamodel will also see the complexity of possible models rise. There is some research being done on how to reduce the size of declarative models [96–98], which could help mitigate the problem. However, it is not yet clear if these techniques are still applicable, and if so, how they would be applied taking into account the introduction of activation decisions and deactivation decisions for constraints. Another possible way to reduce this issue came up during the evaluation, specifically the option to add data-filters to the visualization of a model. This makes it possible to view certain cases in isolation (e.g., clinical pathways), removing all unrelated or inactive constraints from the model.

A third limitation was already discussed in Sect. 2.5.1, namely that the case used in this work had some limitations on the scope. Instead of modeling the complete real-world process of the emergency and orthopedic departments of a hospital, we limited the scope to certain types of arm fractures. This was necessary to reduce the complexity process and its resulting DeciClare model to reasonable levels. As was noted by the domain experts during the evaluation, the added complexity would not have changed anything to the conclusions of this chapter. In the next step of our research project, we are going to use DeciClare to model the whole real-life process in the emergency department of a big Belgian hospital. A final limitation relates to a design decision made in Sect. 2.6.1. Although most of the language very much supports conformance checking, the choice to not have activated constraints apply retroactively can be seen as a small restriction on its conformance checking potential. However, these types of constraints would be very hard to enforce, as process actors would only know in hindsight whether some constraint should have been enforced. So, this concept is not very useful for any sort of active use of process models.

The last limitation relates to the scope of the decision modeling aspect of Deci-Clare. DeciClare focusses on the specific combinations of data values that lead to certain behavior. For example, if a patient has a suspected lower arm fracture then a scan needs to be made. Yet, these data values are just the consequences of an actual decision rationale that was applied. For example, a scan is needed to check if there is indeed a fracture and, if so, to determine the position of the fractured bone endings. The decision rationale is certainly more valuable knowledge. However, a huge time and/or effort investment of the knowledge workers is needed to make these decision rationales explicit. The only options to gather some data on decision rationales is through interviews or by asking the knowledge workers to think aloud during their daily tasks and recording this. The former is often inefficient and incomplete, while the latter is very invasive and difficult to use on a large scale. Nonetheless, including data on the decision rationales would certainly be beneficial when modeling loosely framed KiPs. In the future, an extension of DeciClare could be considered to include this, similar to how this is included in KiPN [99].

The future research plans start with the four limitations discussed above. Additionally, we will study how DeciClare can support simulation techniques and provide a foundation for offering guidance and recommendations to the process workers at run-time.

Research Contributions of Chapter 2

- The metamodel of the Declare process modeling language
- The metamodel of the ConDec-R extension of Declare
- The metamodel of the DeciClare modeling language for loosely frame KiPs
- A classification of (process) modeling languages: multi-perspective and mixed perspective

Chapter 3
Discovering Loosely Framed Knowledge-Intensive Processes Using DeciClareMiner

This chapter is the result of EC4. It describes the development of an automated process and decision discovery technique for loosely framed KiPs.

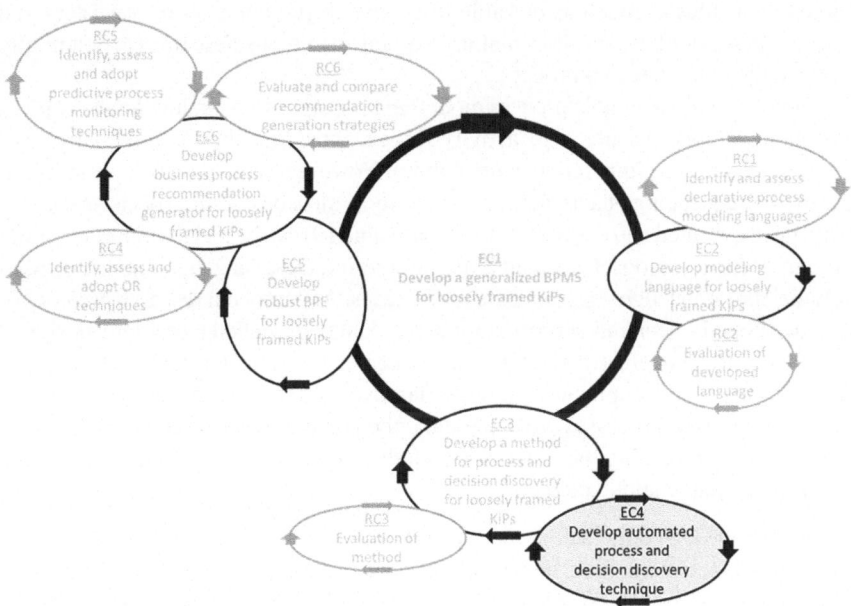

Mertens, S., Gailly, F., Poels, G.: *Discovering healthcare processes using Deci-ClareMiner*. Health Systems. Volume 7, 195–211 (2018) reprinted by permission of the publisher (Taylor & Francis Ltd, http://www.tandfonline.com). https://doi.org/10.1080/20476965.2017.1405876

© Springer Nature Switzerland AG 2020
S. Mertens: Enabling Process Management for Loosely Framed
Knowledge-Intensive Processes, LNBIP 409,
https://doi.org/10.1007/978-3-030-66193-9_3

3.1   Introduction

Business process modeling has been successfully adopted in many different sectors. However, healthcare is one of the few sectors that have yet to fully embrace the process-driven approach [14], even though some of the main concerns trending in eHealth are very similar to those of other sectors, namely, cost reduction, efficiency and patient orientation [100]. The specific characteristics of healthcare processes and, more generally, of loosely framed KiPs are the primary cause [6]. These processes typically have a set of possible activities that can be executed in many different ways, leading to situations where deviations and variations are the norm rather than the exception. The knowledge workers executing a process (e.g., doctors or other healthcare personnel) decide which activities to perform and when they are to be performed. To make these decisions, they often use what is called tacit knowledge: they have an implicit idea of the appropriate actions to perform when certain conditions apply [14]. This idea might be partially based on explicit knowledge (e.g., medical or hospital guidelines), but experience usually factors in heavily. Of course, it would be beneficial for an organization to not only transform these implicit ideas into explicit rules as much as possible to be able to provide a more consistent and transparent service but also allow making explicit changes to these rules to potentially improve the outcomes of a process.

Many currently available process modeling languages focus solely on the explicit sequencing of the activities (e.g., activity X is executed first, then Y, and finally Z) of these processes (i.e., imperative control flow). However, exposing the decisions that govern the sequencing of activities (e.g., activity Y must be executed because activity X has been executed and data attribute 'd' has value 19) can be just as important, if not more important, for loosely framed KiPs. As a result, these languages cannot be used to model the knowledge governing these processes. As part of our research project, we have developed a declarative process modeling language, called DeciClare, designed specifically for modeling these types of processes (see chapter 2). DeciClare uses decision logic as a complement to the declarative modeling concepts to provide the means to describe processes from the data perspective. A new tier of applications is unlocked by modeling the processes with this higher level of detail. Consider the following example applications:

- The knowledge contained by models will make simulations much more realistic and flexible. For example, how would a department address an increase in a group of pathologies by 5%? Would this create new bottlenecks? Can these be eliminated by changing, if possible, some decision criteria?
- The decision logic of certain treatments in models can be compared to the available clinical guidelines. Do the doctors follow the guidelines? If not, what are the characteristic and decision criteria of the cases in which they diverge from the guidelines?
- The knowledge of the mined models can be used to bring interns up to speed quicker or even to educate future nurses/doctors as part of medical courses.

However, the manual creation of decision and process models of real-life loosely framed KiPs remains a problem. Parts of the knowledge that must be captured in these models is typically missing due to its tacit nature. This greatly hinders the adoption of many process modeling, analysis and redesign techniques for loosely framed KiPs. Therefore, the research question addressed by this chapter is as follows: *"How can we automatically and efficiently discover DeciClare models, keeping in mind the computational challenge due to the vast amounts of data that need to be processed in realistic use cases?"*

The process mining domain provides ways to (semi-)automatically discover, monitor and improve real processes by extracting knowledge from the data logged by the IT systems of organizations during their day-to-day operations [11]. A simple example would be a production line company, where the employees execute their daily activities in a strict sequence while the IT system of the company logs the starts and end times of these activities. Process mining techniques can detect this pattern from the logs and automatically compose a process model that reflects the actual process correctly. The DeciClare language can represent the relevant information of loosely framed KiPs, but a corresponding process mining technique for (semi-)automatically discovering these models is currently missing.

In this chapter, we propose a process mining technique called DeciClareMiner that is specifically developed for loosely framed KiPs. This technique can mine a declarative process model and its corresponding decision logic (i.e., a DeciClare model). In essence, it attempts to offer a more complete picture of the (possibly tacit) knowledge found in loosely framed KiPs. This is achieved by mining the rules that have been applied, implicitly and/or explicitly, in past executions of the process, which are contained within a given event log. The two-phase solution strategy used by the miner to efficiently discover the models is the most important contribution of this work. The strategy intelligently aligns an Apriori-inspired phase with a custom genetic algorithm to considerably reduce the vast search space.

The remainder of this chapter is structured as follows. The next section gives an overview of the related literature. In Sect. 3.3, a brief description of the used modeling language is provided. The research methodology that was applied is discussed in Sect. 3.4. This is followed by a description of the proposed algorithm in Sect. 3.5. In Sect. 3.6, the algorithm is evaluated by applying it to a realistic healthcare case and comparing the results to a benchmark for different levels of complexity. Subsequently, the limitations of the presented algorithm are discussed in Sect. 3.7. The last section concludes the chapter and presents directions for future research.

3.2 Related Work

The healthcare domain turned to process management due to the constant pressure to improve the quality of their services while at the same time reducing the associated costs [101]. Processes in healthcare can be classified as either organizational or medical treatment processes [14]. Medical treatment processes can be further categorized as either standard, routine or non-routine processes according to the level of variability and complexity [102]. This work is focused on routine and non-routine medical treatment processes. To manage the variability and complexity of these processes, several approaches have been proposed. For example, Birkmeyer et al. [103] advocated for the enforcement of hospital volume standards for high-risk procedures. The basic idea is that the large-scale repetition makes these hospitals more capable of managing the variability and complexity. However, Gawande stated that relying on process workers' memory alone is not enough when faced with the occasional extreme complexity and specialization of healthcare. He proposed making extensive use of checklists, similar to in the aviation sector, to reduce human mistakes due to forgetfulness [104]. Another important way to manage medical treatment processes is the use of clinical pathways [15, 88, 105, 106], which model the essential steps in the care of patients with specific clinical problems. Traditional business process management [107–112] and modeling techniques [113–118] have also been applied in different healthcare scenarios.

In the process modeling literature, there are two modeling approaches (three when counting hybrid approaches): imperative and declarative modeling. The former approach explicitly models every possible sequence of activities in the process model, while the latter approach models only the rules that determine if a sequence of activities is (in)valid [17]. The latter is preferred when modeling non-standard healthcare processes, as they do not require enumerating the potentially large number of valid process variations [7, 16, 18]. Many process variations are modeled implicitly, allowing the choice of a suitable variation to be made at runtime for each individual process instance (i.e., episode of care).

Checklists are a form of declarative process model, as they state only that each activity on the list needs to be performed and not how or when. However, they offer limited support to process workers regarding in which situations a certain checklist should be used. Early declarative languages, such as Declare [22], tried to improve on this by allowing general relations between possible activities to be described (e.g., if activity X is performed, then activity Y will need to be performed somewhere in the future). This allows for a checklist, of which activities need to be performed, could be performed and should not be performed, at any point during the execution of a process to be created dynamically. DeciClare (see chapter 2) takes this a step further by allowing the models to specify the actual decision logic, if available, regarding the time at which certain activities must be performed, could be performed or should not be performed. In principle, this allows for the dynamic creation of an intelligent checklist that is tailored to a specific situation.

The automated approach of process mining offers an alternative to manually creating healthcare process models, which is hard and tedious work due to the vast amount of domain knowledge that is required. Process mining techniques have been applied to different aspects of healthcare processes in the past [18, 119–126]. However, these applications typically target more standardized processes while using imperative modeling languages as a foundation. Using process mining in combination with declarative modeling languages is actually a relatively new research topic. Maggi et al. [89] were the first to describe an automated declarative process mining approach, called DeclareMiner. Based on automata, it generates and verifies candidate constraints expressed in the Declare language. By choosing the standard Declare language, the authors limited the approach to discovering only rather simple control flow constraints (i.e., no timed, branched, decision-dependent, data or resource constraints). Later work by Maggi et al. [29] introduced a two-phase approach to improve the performance by using an Apriori-based first phase to reduce the search space. Maggi, Dumas, et al. [75] took their approach a step further by adding support for data conditions in a couple of templates of Declare. More recently, a declarative process miner, called TB-MINERful, which can mine branched constraints, was proposed [31]. It introduced subsumption and set dominance, two techniques that have also been implemented in DeciClareMiner to reduce the sizes of the mined models. Schönig et al. [127] also proposed a framework for the discovery of multi-perspective Declare (MP-Declare) models. The work of Schönig et al. focused on an SQL-like on-demand query system. It does not mine a model on its own; rather, an analyst can manually define queries to examine the event log and find useful rules.

DeciClareMiner has the ambitious goal of discovering the declarative control flow of non-standard medical treatment processes, while at the same time also uncovering the medical knowledge governing them. The utilization of Apriori to mine decision-independent rules in the first phase of DeciClareMiner differs slightly from its application in Maggi et al. We moved away from the basic Apriori approach by differentiating between minimal and non-minimal rules. This customization makes it possible to search for decision-independent rules more efficiently in the second phase of DeciClareMiner. The application of data conditions to a couple of templates of Declare in Maggi, Dumas, et al. is similar to the activation decisions of DeciClare, although DeciClare supports them for all templates. The miners themselves essentially differ regarding the use of a heuristic search strategy for the second phase, allowing our technique to scale better with input using increasing amounts of data values, as shown in Sect. 3.6.3. The MP-Declare language is even more comparable to DeciClare: both are multiperspective declarative languages based on Declare, but DeciClare distinguishes itself by its additional support from the resource perspective and deactivation decisions. The MP-Declare mining approach requires a significant amount of domain knowledge from the analyst to define useful queries manually, narrowing the application area compared to the automatic mining approach of DeciClareMiner.

3.3 Modeling Healthcare Processes: DeciClare

The DeciClare language presented in chapter 2 will be used as the process and decision modeling language. Table 3.1 presents the 9 most used constraint templates of DeciClare, each of which is accompanied by an example that illustrates its meaning and parameters. The parameters I and B define the logical operators that can be used in the parameter expressions of the template as a result of branching. The letter used

Table 3.1 DeciClare constraint templates used in chapter 3

Class	Template	Example
Existence	AtLeast(I, n)	AtLeast(Apply bandage or Apply cast, 2): the sum of the occurrences of Apply bandage and the occurrences of Apply cast must be at least 2
	AtMost(B, n)	AtMost(Examine patient and Take X-ray, 3): the number of co-occurrences of Examine patient and Take X-ray must be at most 3
	First(I)	First(Register patient, Examine patient): either Register patient or Examine patient must be executed before any other event can be executed
	Last(I)	Last(Apply sling or Examine patient): either Apply sling or Examine patient must be executed as the final event
Relation	RespondedPresence(B_1, B_2)	RespondedPresence(AtLeast((Take X-ray and Apply sling) or Apply bandage, 1), AtLeast(Examine patient or Perform surgery, 1)): if Take X-ray and Apply sling or just Apply bandage are executed at least once, then Examine patient or Perform surgery must also be executed at least once somewhere in the trace (before, during or after)
	Response(B_1, B_2)	Response(AtLeast((Take X-ray and Apply sling) or Apply bandage, 1), AtLeast(Examine patient or Perform surgery, 1)): if Take X-ray and Apply sling or just Apply bandage are executed at least once, then Examine patient or Perform surgery must also be executed at least once at some time after Take X-ray and Apply sling or after Apply bandage
	ChainResponse(B_1, B_2)	ChainResponse(AtLeast((Take X-ray and Apply sling) or Apply bandage, 1), AtLeast(Examine patient or Perform surgery, 1)): if Take X-ray and Apply sling or just Apply bandage are/is executed at least once, then Examine patient or Perform surgery must also be executed at least once immediately after Take X-ray and Apply sling or after Apply bandage
	Precedence(B_1, B_2)	Precedence(AtLeast((Take X-ray and Apply sling) or Apply bandage, 1), AtLeast(Examine patient or Perform surgery, 1)): Take X-ray and Apply sling or just Apply bandage can be executed only after Examine patient or Perform surgery has already been executed at least once
	ChainPrecedence(B_1, B_2)	ChainPrecedence(AtLeast((Take X-ray and Apply sling) or Apply bandage, 1), AtLeast(Examine patient or Perform surgery, 1)): Take X-ray and Apply sling or just Apply bandage can be executed only immediately after Examine patient or Perform surgery has been executed at least once

refers to the option of using either the inclusive disjunction (I) or both the inclusive disjunction and conjunction (B).

Table 3.1 omits the timing parameters required for each of the templates, with the exception of the untimed RespondedPresence template, to avoid overloading the table. These are two parameters expressing the time interval in which the constraint applies. For example, Response(AtLeast(e1, 1), AtLeast(e2, 1), 2, 7) expresses that if e1 is executed, then e2 must be executed at least once after at least 2 time units and at most 7 time units after e1 was executed. The lower- and upper-bound time parameters are allowed to be 0 and infinity, respectively, making them reduce to the examples presented in Table 3.1.

DeciClare uses concepts from the DMN decision modeling language to express decision logic. This decision logic is used to define when a constraint can be activated and deactivated. Therefore, a constraint does not have to be satisfied until the activation decision evaluates as true (i.e., decision-dependent). The conditions of a decision can consist of any combination of values of the available data attributes, chained using the logical conjunctive and disjunctive operators (e.g., 'a = True' and ('b = False' or 'c = "clavicle"')). When a constraint has a trivial decision (i.e., one that always evaluates as true), it applies generally (i.e., decision-independent). To illustrate the concept of activation decisions, consider the decision-dependent healthcare rule for the reaction to trauma cases with internal bleeding. The rule would consist of a constraint Response(AtLeast(Doctor examination, 1), AtLeast(Surgery, 1), 0, 10) and an activation decision that evaluates as true when it is a trauma case and when the patient exhibits signs of shock and/or heavy local inflammation or pain. This implies that when a patient is a trauma victim and is showing signs of shock and/or heavy local inflammation or pain, surgery must be performed within 10 time units after examination by a doctor. The constraint will be activated during such an examination, prompting emergency surgery.

3.4 Research Methodology

This chapter applies the Design Science Research Methodology [38, 39] to develop a process mining tool (i.e., the design artifact) that can mine a declarative process and decision model from data logged in the information systems of an organization. The requirements for the design artifact are as follows:

- It should be able to handle an event log as input. We will assume that the event log is available as an XES-file. The standard XES should be fully supported, as well as (custom) extensions to add extra data and resource definitions.
- It should offer parameters to handle noise in event log and set the granularity of the output models.
- The output should be a mixed-perspective process and decision model.
- It should be able to run in practical timespans. We defined this as support for 'given an amount of time, give me the best possible model that you can mine'.

The scope is set to the 9 constraint templates from the functional and control-flow perspectives (including negation and branched templates) (see Table 3.1) and activation decisions from the data perspective. These are certainly the most useful and therefore could be regarded as the minimum viable product. Also, most of the data and resource templates of DeciClare cannot be mined automatically using a traditional event log because these logs do not have the ability to store the required data (e.g., the number of instances available of a certain resource at a certain time, authorization templates etc.).

The evaluation will focus on the last two requirements, as the first two are mostly default requirements for any process mining tool. The resulting tool will be compared with a naïve brute-force strategy. The comparison will feature the completeness of the model and the time required to discover it.

3.5   Discovering Healthcare Process Models: DeciClareMiner

The process mining algorithm that can be used to discover DeciClare models is called DeciClareMiner. Figure 3.1 presents a high-level flow diagram of the proposed Deci-ClareMiner algorithm. The input, i.e., an event log, is first entered into the phase 1 algorithm (described in Sect. 3.5.1). In the first phase, all rules that always apply according to the log, independent of decisions, are mined (e.g., AtLeast([Clinical examination of patient], 1)). These rules have a trivial activation decision (i.e., the decision always evaluates as true). The outcome of this phase is twofold: a set of decision-independent rules and a set of rules that did not make the cut but satisfy certain criteria (e.g., Response(AtLeast(Perform surgery, 1), AtLeast(Apply cast, 1)) with a trivial activation decision, is correct for 493 traces and violated in 4018 traces). The former will be stored temporarily pending the completion of the rest of the algorithm. The latter, together with the original event log, will serve as the input for the phase 2 algorithm (described in Sect. 3.5.2). The second phase mines rules that only apply in specific situations and thus are dependent on certain (activation) decisions (e.g., Response(AtLeast(Perform surgery, 1), AtLeast(Apply cast, 1)) acti-vateIf[[Fractured bone = Wrist, More than 16 yrs old = true], [Fractured bone = Wrist, Extensive damage to arteries or nerves = true], [Open or complex fracture = true, Fractured bone = Wrist], [Fractured bone = Forearm], [Fractured bone = Wrist, Periosteum torn = false]]). The outcome of this phase will complement the already mined decision-independent rules with decision-dependent rules to form the eventual outcome of DeciClareMiner: a DeciClare model of the process contained by the given event log (with a given minimal confidence and support level). Table 3.2 presents explanations of important concepts that are used throughout this chapter.

Table 3.2 Explanations of important concepts used in chapter 3

Concept	Explanation
Activity	An identifiable action performed by a process actor as part of achieving a goal of the process. It can consume both time and resources and can produce data
Event	An occurrent of something that happened during the execution of a process. We make a distinction between activity and data events. The former represents the start, end or failure of the execution of an activity by a process actor. The latter represents the moment when a certain data value was made available to the process actors. Resource events are outside of the scope of this project
Trace	Each individual execution of the process as logged by the information system(s) of an organization. It consists of a sequence of activity events performed and the data events that were generated during the execution of the process instance. In healthcare, a trace aligns with what is called an episode of care for one patient
Event log	A collection of many traces relating to the execution of one specific process
Constraint template	A type of constraint (e.g., AtLeast). A template has a specific interpretation and can have certain parameters
Constraint	A (mandatory or optional) limitation of the universe of discourse represented by the process model (e.g., AtLeast(A, 1, 0, 5)). A constraint is an instantiation of a template, with values given for all necessary parameters
Constraint activation	A constraint for which the activation decision evaluates as true and, when it is a relation constraint, the condition side of the constraint is satisfied. This says nothing about the satisfaction of the actual constraint
Conforming activation	A constraint that is activated *and* satisfied by a certain (partial) trace (e.g., consequence side of an activated relation constraint is satisfied)
Violating activation	A constraint that is activated *and* violated by a certain (partial) trace (e.g., consequence side of an activated relation constraint is not satisfied)
Vacuous satisfaction	A constraint that is not activated and thus holds trivially (i.e., it is not violated)
Rule	A constraint in the context of a certain event log. A rule contains a constraint and the corresponding statistics related to the application of the constraint in the given event log (e.g., confidence and support of the constraint)
Conformance percentage (a.k.a. confidence) of a constraint	The number of conforming activations of a rule (i.e., vacuous satisfactions are ignored) divided by the total number of activations of the rule. For example, a rule that has 493 conforming activations and 4018 violating activations has a confidence of 10.9% ($= 493/(493 + 4018)$)

(continued)

Table 3.2 (continued)

Concept	Explanation
Support percentage of a constraint	The total number of traces in which a rule is activated (i.e., vacuous satisfactions are ignored) divided by the total number of traces in the event log. For example, a rule that has 493 conforming activations and 4018 violating activations in a log of 5000 traces has a support of 90.2% (= (493 + 4018)/5000)
Branching level of a constraint	The number of activity/event parameters of most DeciClare constraints can be increased from level 1 (e.g., at least one CT scan must be performed) to higher levels by introducing logical conjunctions and disjunctions (e.g., level 2: at least one echo or CT scan must be performed)
Model fit	How well a model fits the set of given observations. This typically directly correlates to its predictive power for future observations
Overfit	A model that corresponds too closely or exactly to the data used for its creation. It may therefore fail to fit additional data or predict future observations reliably
Underfit	A model that corresponds too little to the data used for its creation. It may therefore fail to encapsulate the logic of the underlying phenomenon with enough details to predict future observations reliable

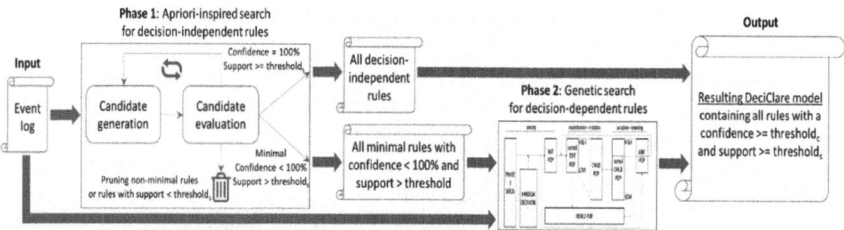

Fig. 3.1 High-level flow diagram of the proposed DeciClareMiner algorithm

3.5.1   Phase 1: Mining Decision-Independent Rules

The algorithm used to mine rules that always apply is largely inspired by the Apriori algorithm [128]. The Apriori algorithm was originally designed to mine frequent itemsets in the context of association rule mining. An itemset is called frequent if it occurs at least a certain number of times (i.e., support is higher than the given threshold). Apriori uses a breadth-first complete-search approach that starts from the smallest frequent itemsets and works its way up to the largest available frequent itemsets. The key principle used by the Apriori algorithm is that any subset of a frequent itemset must also be a frequent itemset. Thus, for example, a set containing items A and B cannot be frequent if either (or both) item A or item B on its own is not frequent. Instead of evaluating every possible combination of items, only those that have a chance of being a frequent itemset are evaluated.

Although declarative rules can be perceived as more complex association rules, identifying declarative rules in an event log is quite different from identifying frequent itemsets in a transactional database. First, the evaluation of a rule is much more complex compared to simply counting occurrences in transactions. Each constraint template has a different logic that needs to be evaluated. Additionally, we are interested in not only the support of a rule in the event log but more so its corresponding confidence. Second, DeciClare does not have only templates connected to one logical expression but also templates that are connected to two logical expressions (i.e., relation templates). Finally, several templates also have an integer parameter (i.e., a bound) in addition to one or two logical expressions. Therefore, to use the Apriori algorithm, a mapping of its core concepts needs to be defined (see Table 3.3). The pseudocode that results from the mapping of the Apriori pseudocode is presented in Table 3.4. In the remainder of this section, the non-trivial mapping steps will be explained in more detail.

3.5.1.1   Leveraged Property

In the mapping of the goal of the algorithm, we introduced the notion of a minimal rule. A rule is minimal if no subset of the connected logical expression results in an equal or lower number of violations. In terms of the goal of the algorithm, discovering a non-minimal rule gets us no closer to a rule with a 100% confidence level than at least one of the previously discovered rules, with a logical expression that is a subset of the non-minimal rule, already did. The non-minimal rule thus offers no additional value over a subset rule that has at most an equal number of violations; at the same time, it is more complex. Consider, for example, an event log with three traces: A, AB and ACD. Evaluating response constraints with only event A in the condition side logical expression results in Fig. 3.2. The first step calculates the confidence level of rules with a consequence-side logical expression size of 1 (e.g., '+1' = one conforming occurrence, and '−2' = two violating occurrences, resulting in a 33% confidence level). In the following step, these are joined pairwise to create rules with a consequence-side logical expression size of 2. Response(AtLeast(A, 1), AtLeast(B or C, 1)) is a minimal rule because it has one less violation than any of its subsets, in this case, than its parent rules Response(AtLeast(A, 1), AtLeast(B, 1)) and Response(AtLeast(A, 1), AtLeast(C, 1)). The same can be said of Response(AtLeast(A, 1), AtLeast(B or D, 1)). However, Response(AtLeast(A, 1), AtLeast(C or D, 1)) is not a minimal rule because it has the same number of violations, namely, 2, as both of its parents

Table 3.3 Mapping of the Apriori algorithm to our problem domain

	Apriori for frequent itemsets	Apriori for declarative rules
Input	A transactional database and a minimal support threshold	An event log, a minimal support threshold and a minimal confidence threshold
Element	Itemsets	Rules connected to logical expressions consisting of activities, events, resources or data elements
Goal	Identify all itemsets with a support level at least equal to a given value (=frequent itemset)	Identify all minimal declarative rules with confidence and support levels at least equal to given values (=frequent minimal rules)
Leveraged property	Any subset of a frequent itemset is also frequent	Any rule connected to a logical expression that is a subset of the logical expression connected to a minimal rule (same template) is also minimal
Iteration principle: initialization	Start from all possible itemsets with size 1	For each type of constraint template, start from constraints with logical expressions of size 1 (i.e., no logical operators)
Iteration principle: joining	Increase the sizes of the itemsets by joining all sets that differ by one element	Increase the size of the connected logical expressions by joining all rules based on the same constraint template that do not have a 100% confidence level and have logical expressions that differ by just one element
Iteration principle: optimization	Only evaluate itemsets that can have a support level at least equal to a given value	Only evaluate rules that can reduce the number of violations while still having a support level at least equal to a given value

Table 3.4 Pseudocode of the first phase of the algorithm

Input: set F_1 containing all minimal rules with logical expressions of size 1, a support threshold, a confidence threshold and a maximal branching level m

Output: set F containing the union of sets F_1, F_2...

For k = 1 to m or until F_k is empty

1. Generate candidates set C_{k+1} containing rules with logical expressions of size k+1 by joining set V_k, which contains all rules in set F_k with at least one violation, with itself
2. Prune C_{k+1} by removing all rules that have a logical expression that contains the logical expression of a non-minimal rule of size k based on the same constraint template
3. Evaluate the rules in C_{k+1}, and put the rules with at least one conforming occurrence into set F_{k+1}

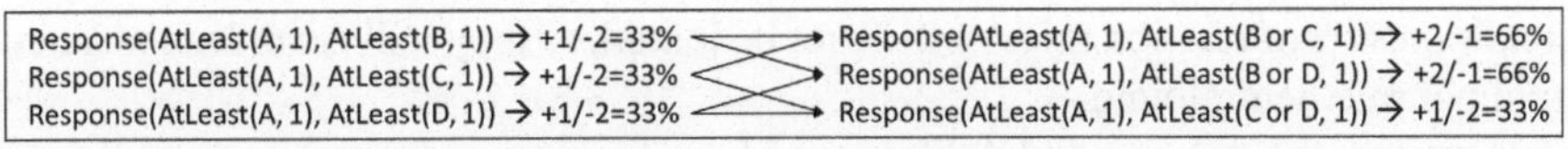

Response(AtLeast(A, 1), AtLeast(B, 1)) → +1/-2=33%	Response(AtLeast(A, 1), AtLeast(B or C, 1)) → +2/-1=66%
Response(AtLeast(A, 1), AtLeast(C, 1)) → +1/-2=33%	Response(AtLeast(A, 1), AtLeast(B or D, 1)) → +2/-1=66%
Response(AtLeast(A, 1), AtLeast(D, 1)) → +1/-2=33%	Response(AtLeast(A, 1), AtLeast(C or D, 1)) → +1/-2=33%

Fig. 3.2 Example of the evaluation of the response template

Response(AtLeast(A, 1), AtLeast(C, 1)) and Response(AtLeast(A, 1), AtLeast(D, 1)). Based on the property of Table 3.3, we can already conclude that the rule Response(AtLeast(A, 1), AtLeast(B or C or D, 1)) is non-minimal, as it contains the non-minimal subset rule Response(AtLeast(A, 1), AtLeast(C or D, 1)).

3.5.1.2 The Iteration Principle: Optimizations

The three steps of the algorithm in Table 3.4 are repeated until the constraints are branched up to the maximal branching level or until no new constraints are found in the previous execution of these steps. The leveraged property allows for three optimizations to be applied in this iteration: the join criteria, the join step and the prune step. The latter does not differ from the corresponding step in Apriori, but the former two require slightly more attention.

3.5.1.3 The Join Criteria

Similar to Apriori, a join can be applied to two rules if the logical expressions differ by exactly one element. However, an additional criteria states that only rules with a confidence level lower than 100% will be joined. This is because joining two rules, of which at least one has a confidence level of 100%, will not result in anything better than the two original rules. For example, joining rules Response(AtLeast(A, 1), AtLeast(B, 1)) and Response(AtLeast(A, 1), AtLeast(C, 1)) will result in a rule Response(AtLeast(A, 1), AtLeast(B or C, 1)), which will be explained below. If it is already known that event A is always followed by event B (confidence level of 100%), then additionally stating that A is always followed by event B or C (i.e., the child rule) offers no new information.

3.5.1.4 The Join Step

Rules with a logical expression of size k are joined to create rules with a logical expression of size k+1 in the iteration steps of the algorithm. However, the elements of the logical expressions can be connected with either the inclusive disjunction or the logical conjunction operator. Therefore, the influence of joining these logical expressions using either operator on the number of violations and the support level is investigated for each template when the leveraged property from Table 3.3 is applied (see Appendix E for the details). As a result, certain rules (e.g., OR join for the condition side of relation rules) will never be joined, as they will never lead to a new minimal rule being found.

However, the AtLeast and AtMost templates have an additional numerical limit associated with them. This makes it very inefficient to apply the Apriori candidate generation step to these templates, as this would require the generation of all possible event sets of size k with all possible limits (= a candidate set of infinite size). Instead, our algorithm makes an exception regarding the Apriori-inspired iteration for these templates and will generate all possible logical expressions and, for each logical expression, calculate the associated limit based on the event log directly. To increase the efficiency, these templates are evaluated together, which makes it possible to generate all rules with a meaningful limit of both templates for some logical expression in one pass of the event log with no performance hit compared to evaluating one rule of these templates (similar optimization is also used for the other templates). For example, suppose A occurs twice and three times, respectively, in an event log with two traces. With a support level of more than 50%, two meaningful rules can be mined in one step: AtLeast(A, 2) and AtMost(A, 3).

3.5.1.5   Running Example

To illustrate how the first phase works, let us consider the following example for the consequence side of the positive Response template (Fig. 3.3). We have an event log of a process with the following traces: AB, AAB, CAC and ABABC. The confidence threshold will be set at 80%, and the support threshold at 50%. The algorithm starts by creating every Response constraint possible with a condition and consequence expression of size 1. The candidates are subsequently evaluated by calculating their confidence and support levels. The first candidate rule has a confidence and support level above the given thresholds and will therefore be added to the result set. Note that the first five rules are minimal rules, as they have no subset rules, but only the first rule is a frequent minimal rule. Next, a new set of candidate rules is generated by joining all compatible candidate rules from the previous candidate set. Joining the consequence side of the positive Response template will be done using only the

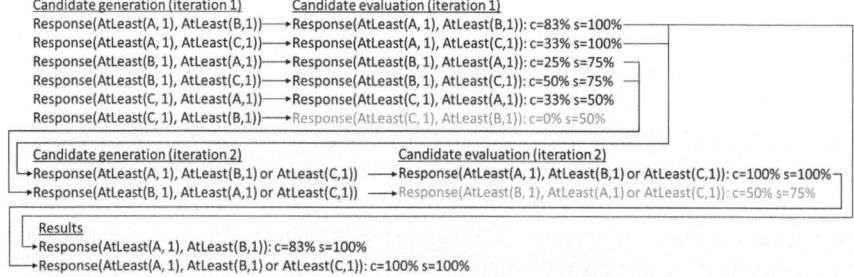

Fig. 3.3 Running example of the first phase (minimal rules in black; non-minimal rules in grey)

OR operator (see Appendix E). Additionally, the last two rules from the candidate set from iteration 1 are not joined since the latter rule has a confidence of 0% (i.e., non-minimal). The result is a new candidate set with two new candidate rules. Since all rules from the candidate set of the previous iteration are minimal, no candidates can be pruned at this point. The subsequent evaluation of the candidates yields one frequent minimal rule and one non-minimal rule (i.e., the second candidate has as many violations as the fourth candidate rule, which is one of the parent rules, from iteration 1). The first candidate will be added to the result set to give us two frequent minimal rules. The algorithm stops at this point, as no candidates of size 3 can be generated.

3.5.1.6 The Output of the First Phase

This first phase results in a set of decision-independent rules with a confidence and support level equal or higher than the given thresholds and logical expressions of a size equal to or less than the given maximal branching level (top output in Fig. 3.1). As a waste product, it also generates all minimal rules no matter the confidence and support levels. This set of 'waste' rules will be used to optimize the second phase of the algorithm (bottom output in Fig. 3.1). With the exception of the AtLeast, AtLeastChoice, AtMost and AtMostChoice templates, all decision-dependent rules can be represented by one of these waste rules combined with some decision. Therefore, the constraints of all these minimal waste rules with a confidence level of less than 100% and a support level higher than the support threshold (as the support level of a rule can only drop by adding an activation decision) that were generated during this first phase will be used as seed constraints for the second phase. In the running example, this would be the first five candidate rules from the first iteration. As a result, the second phase will not have to generate any constraints and can focus on only the decision logic. This will significantly reduce the complexity of defining a search strategy for finding decision-dependent rules and substantially reduce the size of the search space.

For the AtLeast and AtMost templates, only the AtMost rules with 100% confidence levels are used as input, as these express the boundaries within which it is meaningful to search for the decision-dependent rules of these templates. For example, from the rule AtMost(A, 3), with a confidence level of 100%, we can deduce that any meaningful decision-dependent AtMost rule with the same logical expression must have a bound of 0, 1 or 2 and that any meaningful decision-dependent AtLeast rule with the same logical expression must have a bound of 1, 2 or 3.

3.5.2 Phase 2: Mining Decision-Dependent Rules

In the second phase, decision-dependent rules are generated. Our assumption is that for loosely framed KiPs, the number of possible activities will be much lower than the number of possible combinations of data elements on which the activation decisions are based. Therefore, while the first phase uses a complete search algorithm, the second phase uses a heuristic approach to search for meaningful rules from the vast set of possible combinations of data values and seed constraints from the first phase.

For problems with a search space that is too large to go over completely, heuristics can offer 'good enough' solutions by sampling the search space. A subset of these heuristics, called genetic algorithms, mimic evolutionary processes that utilize natural selection. These processes are non-deterministic but have been proven and tested by nature to be very flexible and efficient. The heuristic that we use belongs to the class of genetic algorithms that use the crossover, mutation and selection operators to solve constrained or unconstrained optimization problems [129]. The approach requires the problem to be redefined in terms of finding the best genetic codes (i.e., individuals) according to some fitness function. An individual consists of a subset of the available genes, which are the features that can make the individual a better or worse fit as a solution for a problem compared to other individuals. A population of these individuals is recombined and mutated over multiple iterations to allow the fitness of the population to evolve by sharing the genes of the better individuals. Table 3.5 presents a mapping of the general genetic approach to our problem domain.

The search problem of finding the best decision-dependent rules can be redefined as finding activation decisions for the seed constraints from the first phase. An individual is a combination of a seed constraint and a non-trivial activation decision. The decision values, which can form an activation decision, can be regarded as the genes of the genetic code of individuals. The basic approach is illustrated in Fig. 3.4.

Table 3.5 Mapping of the genetic approach to our problem domain

	Genetic decision-dependent rule miner
Input	Seed rules, the available data elements, an event log, an intermediate population size, a minimal support threshold and a minimal confidence threshold, the number of new seeds to be added in each iteration, a fitness function and a recombination and mutation frequency
Element	A decision-dependent rule, with its activation decision serving as its genetic code
Fitness	A measure of how well a decision-dependent rule reflects the underlying process of the event log
Goal	Find the best decision-dependent rules with a confidence and support above the thresholds
Operations	To find better decision-dependent rules, changes are introduced by recombining and mutating candidates; this allows good decision logic to be shared across the population
Iteration principle	The best decision-dependent rules of the previous iteration and some new seed rules with random decisions form the population of the next iteration; this offers a balance between searching in a specific direction (i.e., of previously found good decision-dependent rules) versus in all directions (i.e., new good decision-dependent rules)

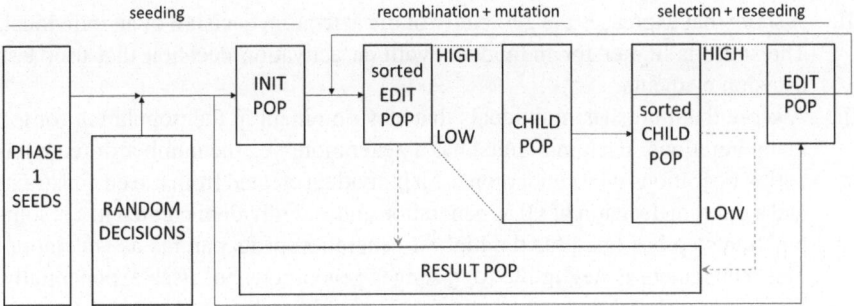

Fig. 3.4 Overview of the second phase of the algorithm

The algorithm starts by combining seed constraints, produced in the first phase, with random activation decisions (e.g., 'Has fever?' = false and 'headache' = true) to create the initial population of individuals. The individuals in the initial population are then evaluated and sorted according to the fitness function. The recombination operator is subsequently used to create a population of children of this population. The higher the fitness of a rule, the higher the chances of being selected as one of the two parent rules of a new child rule. The child gets half of the genes of each parent, with some random mutations being applied to the genes based on the mutation rate. In the next step, this child population is evaluated and sorted according to the fitness function. The best children are used to create a new edit population, together with a given percentage of new seeds in each iteration. This edit population is used to start the next iteration until no new individuals are added to the result population during a given number of iterations or the given maximal amount of search time has been exceeded. Individuals that satisfy the confidence threshold are integrated into the result population during the two evaluation and sort steps of each iteration. Note that the support threshold is ignored at this point and will only be introduced during the post-processing steps, because up to that point each disjunct activation decision for a certain constraint is discovered separately and the support of the constraint can only be calculated by combining all these disjunct pieces into one rule during post-processing.

3.5.2.1 Fitness Function

To measure the fitness of an individual, we use the weighted average of four partial scores (all expressed as percentages):

I. A score that expresses the increase of the trace conformance (i.e., number of conforming traces divided by the total number of traces for which the rule was activated) of an individual compared to the decision-independent seed rule on which the individual was based.

II. A score that expresses the generality of the activation decision of an individual. The score is higher for individuals with an activation decision that uses less decision elements.

III. A score that punishes individuals that stay dominant in the population for too many iterations. Each individual has a generation, i.e., the number of recombination operations it has undergone. An individual created from a seed constraint and a random decision has 0 as generation and an individual created in a recombination step has one plus the highest generation of its parents as generation. The punishment is negligible for younger generations but rises exponentially. This ensures that the search direction stays sufficiently broad.

IV. A score that expresses the potential of the individual to increase the diversity of the result population. A frequency map, which stores the number of times a certain constraint (with its specific parameter values, ignoring the activation decision) has already been found with satisfactory confidence and support levels, is kept. An individual with a constraint that is part of an already found individual will progressively receive a lower and lower score as the frequency of found individuals with the constraint rises. This ensures that other search directions will be explored more frequently as frequent search directions are being exhausted.

3.5.2.2 Optimization

The obvious choice would be to run the second phase algorithm for all templates at once. However, because we grouped certain templates together to increase the efficiency of the evaluation step, the fitness score of such a group of constraints cannot be fairly compared to that of other groups based on other templates. For example, a relation group evaluates the RespondedPresence, Response, ChainResponse, Precedence, and ChainPrecedence templates as well as their negative counterparts for a certain set of required parameters, while the bounded group does the same for the AtLeast and AtMost templates. Its score for the partial fitness measure I is a weighted combination, based on the subsumption hierarchy [97], of the scores of all rules found for this group. However, for the bounded group, there will always be at least one rule found with a confidence of 100% because of how they are evaluated: AtMost(AE, x), with x being the maximum number of times the activity expression 'AE' occurred in any trace of the given log (see end of Sect. 3.5.1). Therefore, the bounded group fitness will generally be higher than the relation group fitness. Hence, the second phase algorithm will be executed separately for each group of templates. The size of the intermediate populations for each group is set relative to the number of available seed rules for that group. Each iteration of the global algorithm for the second phase executes one iteration for each group, unless the group has already converged. Finally, the result populations of each group are merged.

3.5.2.3 Running Example

Figure 3.5 presents a running example of how the second phase would be performed for the AtLeast template (i.e., ignoring the AtMost template of the group). The confidence (c) and support (s) thresholds are set to 100% and 50%, respectively. For simplicity, we set the size of the intermediate populations to just two individuals, with four children, and consider only one seed constraint, namely, AtLeast(A, 1) (i.e., 'A is executed at least once'), with its corresponding decision-independent rule (i.e., AtLeast(A, 1) with a trivial activation decision) having a confidence of 60% and a support of 100%. One can assume that the bound parameter does not change. Three data attributes are used in this example: x (Boolean), y (Boolean) and z (categorical with values: '1', '2' and '3'). In each iteration, one new seed is added to the new edit population.

In the first step of the second phase, an initial population is created by combining the seed constraint with random decisions based on the available data attributes. The constraints in the initial population are then evaluated and added to the edit population, which in turn is sorted according to the fitness function. In the next step, the child population is created by recombining the rules in the sorted edit population with random splits of their genes. This process also introduces random mutations in the genes of the children (grey). The child population is then sorted, with one rule making it into the result population. The best rule of the sorted child population is also transferred to the new edit population for the second iteration, along with a new seed constraint combined with another random decision. The process continues until it converges, or the time limit is reached.

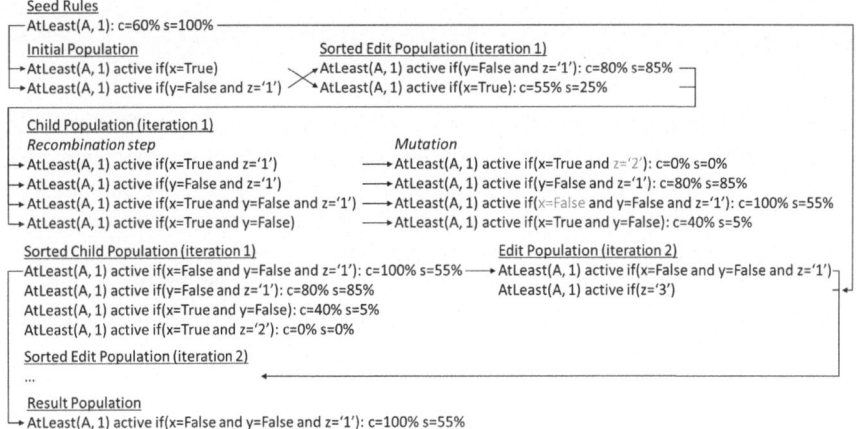

Fig. 3.5 Running example of the second phase

3.5.2.4   The Output After the Second Phase

After the iteration steps of the genetic algorithm, three post-processing steps are performed to improve the combined results from both phases. The first step collects all decision-independent rules that satisfy the confidence and support thresholds from the results of the first phase while also removing subsumed rules according to the subsumption hierarchy (e.g., keep ChainResponse(A, B) and remove Response(A, B), as the former is a stricter version of the latter). The second step merges the decision logic for rules from the results of the second phase with the same constraint but different activation decisions. This step also removes all subsumed rules from these results. The last step combines both results and removes redundant rules (e.g., First(A) makes AtLeast(A, 1) redundant).

3.6   Evaluation

The DeciClareMiner process discovery algorithm is implemented (fully single-treaded) to conduct an evaluation. The implementation of DeciClareMiner used in this chapter can be found at https://github.com/stevmert/DeciClareMinerV11/. The event log and case description (…/models/) as well as a summary of the results of the experiments (…/results/) can also be found at the above link. For the actual results of each of the experiments (ca. 1.13 GB of compressed zip-data, mostly in.CSV format), please contact the author.

3.6.1   Dataset

In the previous chapter, the healthcare process for treating arm-related fractures was modeled using the direct instantiation of the DeciClare abstract syntax metamodel. The process entails the registration, diagnosis and treatment phases for patients with one or more (possible) fractures of a finger, hand, wrist, forearm, upper arm, shoulder, and/or collarbone. This DeciClare process model was created based on the available literature and by interviewing doctors and nurses that participate in this healthcare process in the emergency and orthopedic department of several hospitals in Ghent, Belgium. This fictional (i.e., this is not an isolated process in real-life) but realistic healthcare case will be used for the evaluation of the DeciClareMiner process discovery algorithm.

We first generated an event log based on the DeciClare model of the arm fracture case. We identified 2072 unique realistic combinations of control flow and data that fit the model correctly (i.e., no noise). This is of course a simplification, as the model theoretically allows an infinite number of unique combinations. Additionally, we chose to exclude some of the activities from the original model (i.e., all prescriptions of medication and physiotherapy) for simplicity. The resulting event log uses 9 data attributes, 1 categorical (7 categories) and 8 Boolean, and 9 activities and was created by adding each unique combination of control flow and data at least once, but possibly multiple times (at random), to the log until it contained exactly 5000 traces.

As an example of the kind of rules that correspond to the arm fracture case, consider the following two relatively complex examples. First, one rule yields all situations in which surgery will need to be performed at least once sooner or later: AtLeast(Perform surgery, 1, 0, −1) activateIf[[Open or complex fracture = true], [Fractured bone = Upper arm, No improvement in 3 months = true], [Extensive damage to arteries or nerves = true], [Fractured bone = Upper arm, Both arms broken = true], [Periosteum torn = true, Fractured bone = Wrist]]. The first part represents the constraint (i.e., surgery must be performed at least once), while the second part describes its activation decision (i.e., all the possible data combinations for which the constraint applies). This rule is activated in 4511 of the 5000 traces in the arm fracture event log and thus is regarded as frequent behavior. The second example represents less frequent behavior contained by the event log, i.e., in 493 of the 5000 traces. It describes the situations in which a cast needs to be applied after surgery is performed: Response(AtLeast(Perform surgery, 1, 0, −1), AtLeast(Apply cast, 1, 0, −1), 0, −1) activateIf[[More than 16 yrs old = true, Fractured bone = Wrist], [Extensive damage to arteries or nerves = true, Fractured bone = Wrist], [Open or complex fracture = true, Fractured bone = Wrist], [Fractured bone = Forearm], [Periosteum torn = false, Fractured bone = Wrist]]. The decision logic associated with both of these example rules is presented in its most general and precise form. Of course, subsets of this decision logic exist that describe only parts of the general behavior (i.e., missing disjunctive decision logic or overfitting in a few specific cases) and can therefore uniquely identify only a subset of the traces of these rules.

3.6.2 Benchmark Creation

To analyze the DeciClare models mined using DeciClareMiner, benchmarks were created for several branching levels. A complete search algorithm was used to mine reference models that could serve as benchmarks for branching levels 1 and 3 and for unlimited branching. Table 3.6 highlights some important numbers from the

Table 3.6 Application of the complete search algorithm for different branching levels

Branching level	Time	# of seed rules for Phase 2	# of rules mined in Phase 2	Total # of rules mined in both Phase 1 and 2
1	49 h 39 min	56	129	268
3	353 h 24 min	412	973	1177
Unlimited	734 h 42 min	826	3989	4205

application of the complete search algorithm, which were executed one by one on a single core of an Intel E5-2680v3 with the confidence threshold set to 100% (as there is no noise in the log) and no support threshold (as most of the 2072 variations occur only once or twice due to limiting the log to 5000 traces). From here on, we will refer to the models mined with the complete search algorithm as the 'complete models'. These models do not contain any subsumed or redundant rules, as these are filtered out automatically. Note that the complete model with unlimited branching is not the same as the model from the previous chapter, because the complete model is based on an event log containing just a subset of the behavior of the original model. Each seed rule needed to be checked for all 279935 possible data combinations for both branching levels. This vast search space is the result of the 9 data attributes used in the arm fracture event log and is still very limited compared to real-life cases. Compared to branching level 1, the search space increases by an additional 736% for a branching level of 3 and by 1475% for unlimited branching. This supports the assumption made at the start of Sect. 3.5.2, based on which a heuristic for the second phase of the algorithm was adopted instead of a complete search approach. The increased search space for branching levels higher than 1 make it infeasible to calculate a complete search model in real-life cases.

To calculate how the models mined using DeciClareMiner stack up to the benchmarks, two criteria are used: the percentage of traces uniquely identified, and the percentage of constraints identified by the model as a whole compared to the corresponding reference model. For example, an overfitted version of the first example rule from Sect. 3.6.1 might only be able to uniquely identify 3000 traces. This means that for this rule, the mined model would score 3000 out of a possible 4511 for the first criteria and 1 out of 1 for the second criteria. However, if the mined model does not contain any version of this rule, it would score 0 out of a possible 4511 for the first criteria and 0 out of 1 for the second criteria for this rule. The scores are calculated for each rule in the corresponding reference model, are compared to the rules in the mined model, and together serve as the score for the mined model.

3.6.3   Results

Using the arm fracture case event log as input, DeciClareMiner was executed using the same single core of an Intel E5-2680v3 with the same confidence and support thresholds as for the benchmark creation (100% and 0%, respectively), with different settings for the branching level and amount of search time for the second phase. For each branching level and search time combination, DeciClareMiner was executed many times (i.e., # of experiments column in Table 3.7). This was necessary because the second phase of the algorithm is not deterministic, which means that the results of the miner can vary. Based on many runs of the miner on the same settings, we were able to calculate the average coverage of the mined models using the predefined branching level and search time.

Table 3.7 Results from the mining experiments for different settings

Branching level	Search time P2	% of traces identified	% of constraints identified	# of experiments	Speed-up factor
1	10 min	93.32% ($\sigma = 1.42\%$)	98.72% ($\sigma = 0.84\%$)	271	278
	20 min	97.64% ($\sigma = 0.52\%$)	99.56% ($\sigma = 0.48\%$)	409	145
	40 min	99.05% ($\sigma = 0.19\%$)	99.82% ($\sigma = 0.34\%$)	117	74
3	10 min	69.22% ($\sigma = 1.13\%$)	81.38% ($\sigma = 1.27\%$)	270	1466
	20 min	78.32% ($\sigma = 1.71\%$)	89.39% ($\sigma = 1.28\%$)	410	830
	40 min	87.29% ($\sigma = 1.15\%$)	94.33% ($\sigma = 0.70\%$)	117	462
Unlimited	10 min	50.57% ($\sigma = 1.22\%$)	58.89% ($\sigma = 1.23\%$)	364	2229
	20 min	59.55% ($\sigma = 1.59\%$)	67.85% ($\sigma = 1.78\%$)	572	1312
	40 min	68.2% ($\sigma = 1.04\%$)	77.41% ($\sigma = 1.16\%$)	307	752

The power of the chosen heuristic is illustrated by the fact that DeciClareMiner found 99% of all the constraints and 93% of the total decision logic in just 10 min (see Table 3.7). The benchmark needed 49 h and 38 min to calculate the complete search model. If we assume that the complete search algorithm mined the results evenly over this runtime (i.e., 0.03% per minute), it would have mined 93.32% of the total decision logic after 46 h and 20 min. Then, DeciClareMiner speeds this up by a factor of 277 (i.e., 9.33% per minute). Figure 3.6 illustrates how the intermediate populations evolve during the execution of the algorithm (please note that the results in Fig. 3.6 are a bit worse than the actual performance of the algorithm due to the added overhead of having to store the intermediate population after each iteration). The second phase of DeciClareMiner does most of the work early on due to the innate characteristics of the genetic approach. After just 13 iterations (~1 min), 88% of all the constraints and 61% of the total decision logic had already been found. The scores further approach the model solution with each additional iteration, though the speed drops significantly at the same time. Almost 60% of the model had already been found during the first minute of execution (speed-up factor of 1740). However, although the results further improve with a longer runtime, to 98% and 99% for 20 and 40 min, respectively, the speed-up factor drops significantly at the same time to 145 (4.88% per minute) and 74 (2.48% per minute), respectively.

For branching levels 3 and unlimited branching, the mined models still obtain respectable averages of 87% and 68% of the benchmark model in 40 min. Although the absolute speed declines for higher branching levels (2.18% and 1.70% per minute, respectively, during the 40-min search), the relative speed-up factor remains high compared to the runtimes for a complete search approach. DeciClareMiner speeds up the discovery of 87% of the model by a factor of 462 for branching level 3 and of 68% of the model by a factor of 752 for unlimited branching.

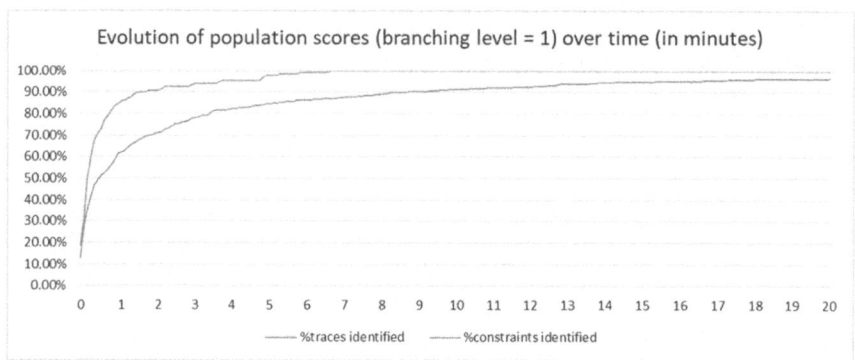

Fig. 3.6 Evolution of the intermediate population scores

3.6.4 Discussion

As illustrated in the evaluation, the miner presented in this work is a promising step towards modeling and capturing the knowledge of real-life healthcare processes and, more generally, of loosely framed KiPs. DeciClareMiner can efficiently mine declarative process models containing decision-independent and decision-dependent constraints. It was able to produce a model that represents 93% of episodes of care with atomic constraints in a relatively short time (10 min). This is considered a major improvement compared to the 50 h it took to calculate the 100%-episode model using an exhaustive search approach. The main building blocks of the DeciClareMiner algorithm, i.e., the Apriori-inspired first phase algorithm and the genetic algorithm of the second phase, can address rising complexity very well. This behavior was expected due to the selection of a genetic algorithm as the basis for the second phase. Similar to the natural processes on which genetic algorithms are based, genetic algorithms offer good performance when faced with high complexity. In addition, although not a part of this evaluation, they should also be able to handle varying levels of noise in the event log, as these techniques are considered relatively noise-resistant.

The downside of using a heuristic to search for decision-dependent rules is that we cannot guarantee that every detail of the complete search model will ever be found. As Fig. 3.6 shows, the algorithm will quickly find most of the complete search model but eventually slows down more and more as it approaches 100%. We believe that this is a necessary trade-off to apply this kind of technique to the domain of healthcare in real-life environments. The calculation time of the unbranched complete model of the arm fracture log already required more than 30 days of nonstop mining. In real-life settings, the cases are much more complex. The event log used in the evaluation has a size of just 26 MB, whereas event logs for real-life cases can easily be hundreds of MB (e.g., the MIMIC-III clinical database contains 43 GB of data [130]). Clearly, the available processing power and time are going to be the limiting factors. Additionally, the domain is very dynamic, as medical knowledge evolves continuously. In this setting, it is better to have a very good approximation of the complete search model in reasonable time than a complete search model that is already at least partially obsolete by the time it is available. We believe that the efficiency offered by DeciClareMiner is necessary for the adoption of process mining in real-life healthcare organizations and, more specifically, in non-standard medical treatment processes.

DeciClareMiner can also be applied when the event log is not complete, as in our evaluation and in almost every practical case. However, this requires a subsequent evaluation of the resulting set of rules by domain experts to relax possibly over-fitted rules. Because DeciClareMiner calculates the whole subsumption hierarchy, this relaxation is just a matter of selecting an already available rule that is lower in the hierarchy (e.g., if the event log only contains episodes of care that execute activity B immediately after A, which is not that strict in real life, the mined rule ChainResponse(A, B) can be relaxed to Response(A, B)). The use of a declarative language makes the evaluation of the rules by domain experts relatively easy, as each rule can be evaluated in isolation.

The availability of DeciClare models of loosely framed KiPs can enable many new applications at the management level. For example, consider the checklists mentioned in Sect. 3.2. They are already being used throughout the healthcare sector at an operational level to reduce the number of human errors that occur due to the innate and overwhelming complexity of non-standard medical treatment processes. Declarative process models can be used to generate these checklists on-demand during the execution of a process. The dynamic checklists can give an overview of the activities that still need to be performed, those that should not be performed and those that are optional. The decision logic in a mined DeciClare model can help produce tailor-made checklists for patients currently being treated, taking into account the specific patient characteristics and progression of treatment. Of course, it would be advisable to have the mined model validated by experts first. The treating physicians could also perform this validation on-the-fly, as the knowledge mined by DeciClareMiner represents only a small portion of their extensive domain knowledge.

3.7 Limitations

The current implementation is already rather efficient, as the first phase and each iteration of the second phase of the algorithm each have a linear asymptotic time complexity (i.e., $O(n)$) in relation to the number of traces in the given event log. However, it should still be considered a proof of concept. There is still significant room for optimization (e.g., better parameter tuning and the introduction of advanced techniques such as parallelization and caching). Additionally, the DeciClare language support will need to be expanded for future use. First, the current implementation can mine nine of the available templates (e.g., no data constraint templates). These nine are considered the most important templates (e.g., most used in the arm fracture model that was made manually in chapter 2). Support for other templates will be added in the future, although some templates cannot be mined automatically (e.g., authorization templates), and several others require information that is not typically available in an event log. Second, the implementation only supports relation templates using the 'at least once' interpretation for the logical expressions of the condition and consequence sides of the constraints (e.g., if A is executed at least once, then B must be executed at least once) and the 'at most zero times' interpretation for the logical expression of the consequence side (e.g., if A is executed at least once, then B can be executed at most zero times). This is similar to the interpretation of the corresponding branched templates in Declare for the positive and negative versions of the relation templates. Third, DeciClare allows constraints to be not only activated by way of a decision but also deactivated. However, from experience, we know that deactivations are required much less frequently compared to activations; thus, including these in the second phase in a similar way would not be very efficient. How to add support for constraint deactivations is still an open research question and might require the introduction of a third phase. Fourth, the current implementation only supports data attributes with a finite domain. A data attribute can have a Boolean (no overlap) or categorical (allowed to overlap) domain, but continuous data attributes (e.g., temperature $= 39.6°$) have not yet been considered. These present a tougher challenge, as it is difficult to process their infinite domains efficiently. An extra preprocessing step by a domain expert is currently required to convert infinite domains to well-defined finite domains until support for these types of data attributes is added. Lastly, the time parameters present in many of the constraint templates are not yet supported. These were included in a previous version of the miner but were only outlined by the minimal and maximal time parameters for each rule and not mined actively. However, this subject will also be revisited as part of future research.

It is also worth noting that the current lack of a visual syntax for DeciClare does not greatly impact DeciClareMiner. When a real concrete syntax becomes available, no changes to the miner itself are required. A visual representation of the mined model can be easily created separately, as the results of DeciClareMiner are a direct instantiation of the abstract syntax of the language, which will have to be the foundation of the visual syntax anyway.

3.8 Conclusions and Directions for Future Research

In this chapter, we proposed a process discovery approach for loosely framed KiPs. The process discovery algorithm of DeciClareMiner can mine DeciClare process models in the form of decision-independent and decision-dependent rules. The algorithm attempts to automatically extract a complete picture of the (possibly tacit) knowledge of a process contained within a given event log.

The algorithm consists of two phases to mine both decision-independent rules and decision-dependent rules. The first phase involves a complete search algorithm inspired by the Apriori association rule mining algorithm, while the second phase involves a heuristic belonging to the class of genetic algorithms. This difference in approach is rooted in the assumption that in the context of loosely framed KiPs, the number of possible activities will be much lower than the number of combinations of available data elements on which decisions are based. This means that using a complete-search algorithm for the first phase is acceptable, while for the second phase, a heuristic is more appropriate. This assumption was confirmed in several healthcare event logs[1]. Although the concept of mining decision-dependent rules is the main contribution of this work, the alignment of the strategies for mining decision-independent and decision-dependent rules is also a novelty. By using the waste generated in the first phase, we can turn the second phase into a much more targeted search. The process discovery algorithm was evaluated using a realistic event log of an arm fracture healthcare process and by comparing the results to a benchmark set obtained via an exhaustive search approach. DeciClareMiner considerably speeds up the discovery of a process model compared to a complete search algorithm. A trade-off was made to prioritize good results in reasonable time over a guaranteed complete model. This makes DeciClareMiner more applicable to real-life scenarios, where time and processing power are limited.

In future research, we will first expand the support of DeciClareMiner for the Deci-Clare language. Section 3.7 reports a number of limitations regarding this support, each of which must be resolved. Additionally, a visualization layer will need to be added when a visual syntax for DeciClare becomes available. The performance of the miner with event logs containing noise will also need to be investigated. Deci-ClareMiner should theoretically be able to successfully handle the presence of noise in event logs, as stated in Sect. 3.6. Nevertheless, this work does not evaluate this property. The main questions are related to the impact of noise on the efficiency of the miner.

RESEARCH CONTRIBUTION OF CHAPTER 3
The process discovery algorithm DeciClareMiner, which can automatically mine a DeciClare model from a given process event log.

---

[1] For the arm fracture event log: 9 activities and 21 data values, leading to 511 activity combinations and ~ 280.000 data combinations

For the Sepsis event log (see §5.2.6.1.1): 16 activities and 214 data values, leading to 65535 activity combinations and ~3*1064 data combinations

For the emergency department event log (see §5.2.6.1.1): 116 activities and 951 data values, leading to ~2*1034 activity combinations and ~2*10286 data combinations

Chapter 4
Integrated Declarative Process and Decision Discovery of the Emergency Care Process

This chapter is the result of EC3. It describes the development of a method for creating a process and decision knowledge base for loosely framed KiPs. The ADR-cycle combines the development of this method with the application of the process and decision discovery technique on real data from the emergency medicine department of a hospital (RC3).

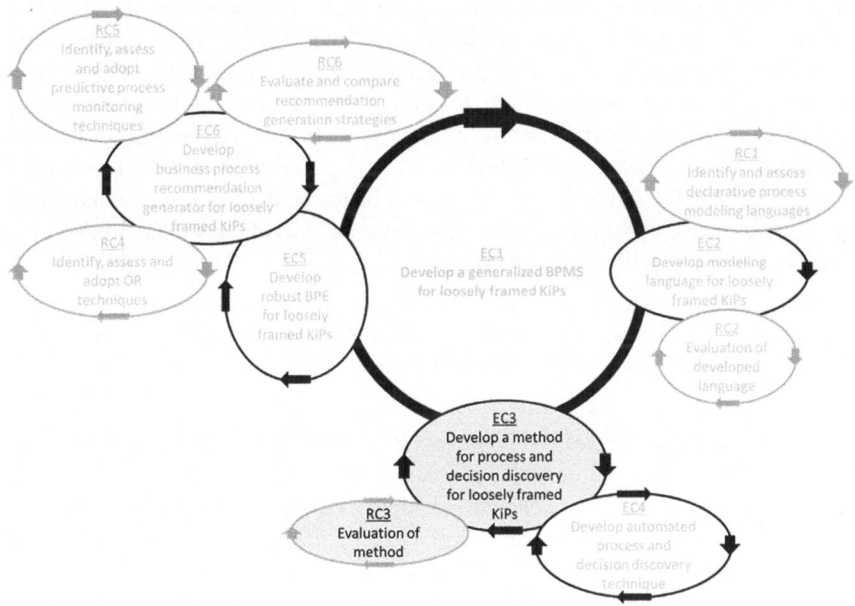

Mertens, S., Gailly, F., Van Sassenbroeck, D., Poels, G.: Integrated Declarative Process and Decision Discovery of the Emergency Care Process. Information Systems Frontiers (2020).
https://doi.org/10.1007/s10796-020-10078-5

4.1   Introduction

Within the Information Systems domain it is generally accepted that a process-oriented approach centered around process modeling results in efficiency gains, efficacy gains and/or cost reduction [131]. Typical examples are applications in sectors such as manufacturing [132], sales [133] and software development [134]. However, the healthcare sector is one the exceptions [14, 135]. This is surprising because some of the main concerns trending in eHealth are very similar to those of these other sectors, namely, cost reduction, efficiency and patient orientation [100]. Healthcare processes can be subdivided in two groups of processes: medical diagnosis/treatment processes and organizational/administrative processes [14]. The slow adoption of process modeling in healthcare is primarily manifested for the medical diagnosis and treatment processes. These processes typically represent the extreme end of the complexity spectrum for processes, hypercomplexity [136], and can be characterized as dynamic, multi-disciplinary, loosely framed, human-centric and knowledge-intensive processes [34, 137]. Loosely framed processes have an average to large set of possible activities that can be executed in many different sequences [6], leading to situations where deviations and variations are the norm rather than the exception [138]. The knowledge workers participating in the execution of a process (i.e., physicians and other healthcare personnel) use cognitive processes to decide which activities to perform and when they are to be performed [139]. To make these decisions, they often leverage what is called tacit knowledge, meaning that they have an implicit idea of the appropriate actions to perform when certain conditions apply [14]. This idea might be partially based on explicit knowledge (e.g., medical or hospital guidelines) but experience usually factors in heavily. This kind of tacit knowledge is also collective in the sense that it often cannot be traced back to just one individual, but rather is (unevenly) spread across organizational units of knowledge workers that share the same or similar experiences [140].

> *"To make medical knowledge broadly available, medical experts need to externalize their tacit knowledge. Thus, improving healthcare processes has a lot to do with stimulating and managing the knowledge conversion processes."*

- Lenz & Reichert (p. 44) [14]

Modeling these processes can be beneficial in many ways. A process model can serve as a means to document the process (which increases transparency for all stakeholders), to communicate changes explicitly, educate students and new process actors, to offer passive process support (i.e., using the model as a roadmap during execution) and as a foundation for active process support and monitoring (e.g., in process engines) and all sorts of management and analysis techniques (e.g., bottlenecks, process improvement...). Process modeling in healthcare has traditionally focused on clinical pathways (CPs) (a.k.a. clinical guidelines, critical pathways, integrated care pathways or care maps) [88, 105, 106, 141–146]. Although the exact definition of what they entail can vary from paper to paper [15], the general consensus seems to be that they are best practice schedules of medical and nursing procedures for the treatment of patients with a specific pathology (e.g., breast cancer). CPs can be considered process models, but they have serious drawbacks. CPs are the result of Evidence Based Medicine, which averages global evidence gathered from exogenous populations that may not always be relevant to local circumstances [147]. Therefore, CPs can be great general guidelines, but real-life situations are typically more complex. Second, comorbidities and practical limitations (e.g., resource availability) can prevent CPs from being implemented as-is. Third, the real process also comprises more than just the treatment of patients, as steps like arriving at a diagnosis and other practicalities should to be considered as well. A CP is therefore a form of high-level model of one idealized process variation. To unlock the full aforementioned benefits, a more complete view on the real processes is needed that encapsulates all possible care episodes within a certain real-life management scope (e.g., department). Of course, CPs and other medical guidelines can subsequently be used to verify whether such model of the real process follows the medical best practices as closely as possible.

Modeling healthcare processes manually, for example by way of interviewing the participants, can be a tedious task due to their intrinsic complexity and the extensive medical knowledge involved. This often leads to a model that paints an idealized picture of the process that overly simplifies reality [148]. Meanwhile, hospital information systems already record a lot of data about these processes for the sake of documentation [149]. The sheer amount of data in these systems makes manual analysis unrealistic. Consequently, there has been an increased interest into process mining techniques that can automate the discovery of healthcare process models from such data sources [125, 150, 159, 160, 151–158] and recent literature reviews indicate that it is still trending upwards [122, 161–163]. However, the existing work is almost exclusively focused on techniques that result in either imperative process models or CPs. The introduction of new process modeling languages based on the declarative paradigm [22, 164] opens up new research avenues [165]. Declarative languages are better suited to represent loosely framed processes because they can model the rules describing the process variations instead of having to exhaustively enumerate all variations as imperative techniques do. The knowledge-intensive side of the processes can be supported by integrating a knowledge perspective into the declarative process modeling languages [127, 137, 166–168]. This allows for the decision logic of the process to be modeled and makes the resulting group of languages a natural fit for loosely framed knowledge-intensive healthcare processes. Declarative process mining techniques have been applied before on healthcare processes, but not on the complete medical care process (e.g., only the treatment of already diagnosed breast cancer patients) [75] and without considering the decision logic that governs the process [18, 169].

From a methodological perspective, methods for the application of data mining have been developed and are widely used [170, 171]. However, these are too high-level and provide little guidance for process mining specific activities [10]. Therefore, methods were developed specifically for the process mining subdomain [34, 35, 160]. These provide a good foundation for typical process mining applications but are geared towards imperative process mining techniques and ignore data and decision aspects of the process. The method of Rebuge and Ferreira [34] is positioned to target healthcare processes, but the use of imperative process mining techniques means that they have to resort to clustering techniques in an effort to filter out some behavior and isolate smaller parts of the process. [34] also represent the method as a straightforward linear approach, which is unrealistic in the context of real-life applications on loosely framed processes.

This chapter reports on an Action Design Research cycle, which is part of the overarching Design Science project to develop a process-oriented system that manages and supports loosely framed knowledge-intensive processes. The research artifact presented in this chapter is a method for process and decision discovery of loosely framed knowledge-intensive processes. This method consists of the preparation of process data to serve as input for a decision-aware declarative process mining tool called DeciClareMiner (see chapter 3), the actual use of this tool and the feedback loops that are necessary to obtain a satisfactory model of a given process. The method was iteratively improved and validated by applying it to a real-life case of an emergency care process.

The remainder of this chapter is structured as follows. Section 4.2 presents our research methodology. Section 4.3 describes the method for process and decision discovery of loosely framed knowledge-intensive processes. The method application is summarized in Sect. 4.4. And finally, Sect. 4.5 concludes the chapter and presents directions for future research.

4.2   Research Methodology

Action Design Research (ADR) [42] is a specific type of Design Science Research [38]. While typical Design Science Research focusses solely on the design of research artifacts that explicitly provide theoretical contributions to the academic knowledge base, ADR simultaneously tries to solve a practical problem [42]. The practical problem serves as a proving ground for the proposed artifact and a source for immediate feedback related to its application. Based on this feedback, the design artifact is iteratively improved. In this paper, the research artifact and practical problem are, respectively, the method for process and decision discovery of loosely framed knowledge-intensive processes and the creation of a process and decision model of a real-life emergency care process.

An ADR-cycle consists of four stages:

Stage 1:   Problem formulation
Stage 2:   Building, intervention and evaluation
Stage 3:   Reflection and learning
Stage 4:   Formalization of learning

The previous section discussed the problem statement: the lack of a process mining method for declarative process and decision mining techniques. Therefore, the research artifact of this paper is a method for process and decision discovery of loosely framed knowledge-intensive processes. This method should consist of the preparation of process data to serve as input for a decision-aware declarative process mining tool, the actual use of this tool and the feedback loops that are necessary to obtain a satisfactory model of a given process.

For the second stage, we have performed an IT-dominant building, intervention and evaluation stage, which is suited for innovative technological design. This stage consists of building of the IT-artifact (i.e., the envisioned method), an intervention in a target organization (i.e., an emergency medicine department), and an evaluation. We started from the existing methods [34, 35] to identify relevant steps in a process mining project. These activities were subsequently evaluated for their applicability to a declarative setting. As the artifact is still in preliminary development, we have limited the repeated intervention steps to light-weight interventions in a limited organizational context [42].

The research artifact was evaluated after each execution of the second stage. The evaluation was performed by the researchers in close cooperation with the head of the emergency medicine department of the hospital. It consisted of two parts, each of which highlighted a different use case of the artifact. The head of the emergency medicine department took on the role of the domain expert, who could identify problems with the application of the research artifact which, in turn, were traced back to the research artifact itself by the researchers. A discussion of the results of the evaluation followed. Potential changes to the research artifact in the context of the practical application were proposed in the first half of these discussions, which corresponds to the reflection and learning stage of the ADR-cycle (i.e., stage 3). The proposed changes were then discussed in the more general context of process and decision mining projects for loosely framed knowledge-intensive processes in the second half of these discussions, which corresponds to the formalization of learning stage of the ADR-cycle (i.e., stage 4). Finally, the resulting changes were implemented to end each iteration of the ADR-cycle. A new iteration was initiated if significant changes were made to the artifact during the previous iteration.

4.3 Discovering the Emergency Care Process with DeciClareMiner

We first created an initial method by combining elements from the existing process mining methods [34, 35] and adapting them to a declarative process mining context (Fig. 4.1). Note that we did not include a process analysis, improvement or support step (as in PM^2 of van Eck et al.). This is because we see these more as separate usage scenarios of the results of process discovery (i.e., the created event log and process model). Such usage scenarios could be part of more general process mining method(ologie)s, but our focus was solely on a method for process discovery [1]. The internal structure or language (grey text) of the inputs and outputs (gold) as well as the entity responsible for the execution (blue text) of each step (green) have also been added. Optional activities are represented by transparent and dashed rectangles.

Table 4.1 Explanations of some of the terminology used in this chapter (also see Table 12)

Term	Explanation
Declarative constraint	A limitation of the allowed behavior when executing a process. This can be both in a positive manner (i.e., a certain activity or event is required to be executed at least a given number of times during a certain time span) and negative manner (i.e., a certain activity or event is prohibited to be executed during a certain time span). The types of constraints can be classified according to the perspective to be modeled: functional/control-flow, data and resource constraints. In this paper we will treat existence (e.g., aforementioned positive and negative examples) and relational constraints (i.e., Response(A, B) states that if A is executed, then B must to be executed somewhere in the future before the process execution ends) as reflecting the functional/control-flow perspective
Data attribute	The definition of some data property in the form of a name and a data type (e.g., the Boolean 'hasPaid?')
Data value	A specific value that a certain data attribute can have (e.g., TRUE)
(De)activation decision	A set of data values connected with logical operators (i.e., AND/OR) that represent a specific process context. For example, certain behavior might apply when the patient is diagnosed with hypothermia or when the patient is alcohol intoxicated and cold (written as [[hypothermia], [alcohol intoxication, cold]] in DeciClare)
Decision-independent constraint	A constraint that has a trivial (i.e., always true) activation decision. This means that there are no data conditions that need to apply for the constraint to be active. Therefore, this kind of constraints must always be satisfied by a process execution. For example, 'Patient registration' must be executed at least once. Note that this term only refers to the data conditions of the activation decision. A relational constraint can have both an activation decision based on data conditions and a specific activity or event (e.g., A in Response(A, B)) that must have occurred before the target becomes required (e.g., B in Response(A, B))
Decision-dependent constraint	A constraint that does not have to be satisfied until the activation decision evaluates as true. It needs to be satisfied starting from when it was activated up until it (optionally) gets deactivated when the deactivation decision evaluates as true. An inactive constraint can be violated with no consequences. For example, the constraint 'after an examination by a physician, surgery has to be performed at least once' and an activation decision that evaluates as true when it is a trauma case and when the patient exhibits signs of shock and/or heavy local inflammation or pain during the examination

(continued)

Table 4.1 (continued)

Term	Explanation
Seed constraint	A decision-independent constraint that has more than enough support but insufficient confidence. For example, Response(A, B) states that if A is executed, then B must be executed at least once somewhere after A. Let us assume minimal support and confidence levels of 10% and 90%, respectively, that A occurs in 15% of the traces of the given event log (i.e., a support level of 15%) and that in 80% of those traces A was eventually followed by B (i.e., a confidence level of 80%). The example constraint is a seed constraint. Adding an activation decision to this seed constraint can result in a constraint with a higher confidence level and a (slightly) lower support level, because it only applies to a subset of the original traces

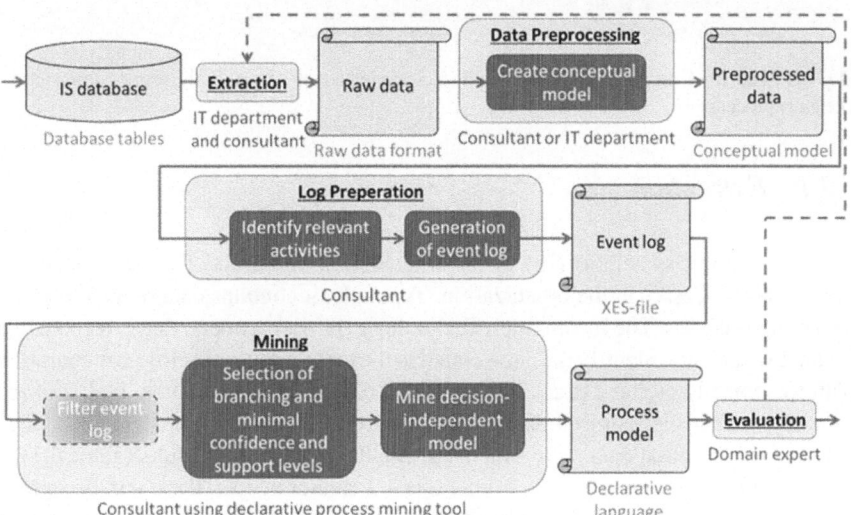

Fig. 4.1 The initial method for process discovery based on existing methods

During different iterations of the ADR-cycle, several missing intermediate activities and iteration loops were identified that were needed to discover a satisfactory process and decision model. The result is presented in Fig. 4.2. The remainder of this section describes each separate step of the method and the intermediate activities they entail.

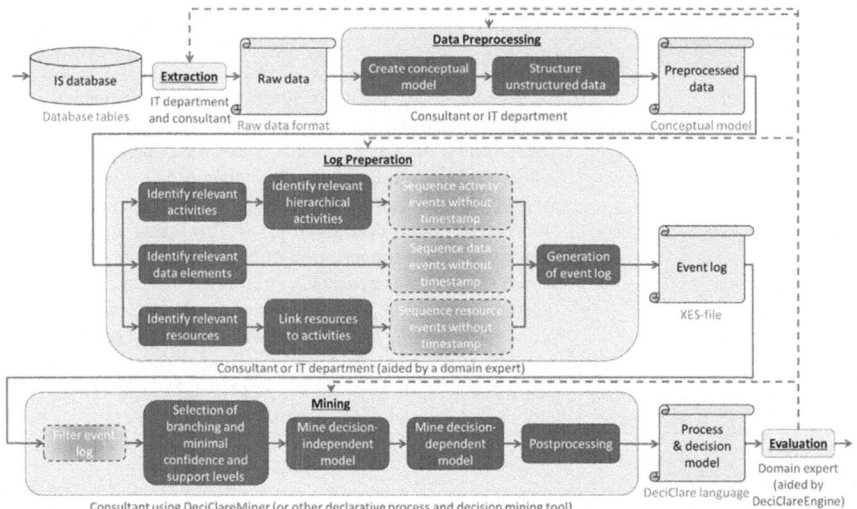

Fig. 4.2 The final method for process and decision discovery for loosely framed knowledge-intensive processes

4.3.1 Extraction

The information system(s) (IS) of an organization contain(s) the data needed to execute all processes in the organization. Typically, it contains data related to many different processes. The Information Technology (IT) department, that is responsible for the IS, must first identify the data related to the target process in close collaboration with the consultant and extract it from the IS database(s). Of course, that is in the assumption that the required data is being stored. Table 4.2 summarizes the ideal data and the minimal data requirements to enable high-quality results (Table 4.1).

If the minimum requirements from Table 4.2 cannot be met, there will be significant limitations to the results of the method application. This will often be the case in real-life applications with data sources that are process-unaware (i.e., systems that are oblivious to the process context in which data processing takes place) [1]. Typical issues include missing events and inaccurate timestamps (e.g., the stored timestamp corresponds to when the data is entered in the system but deviates from when the activity actually took place). However, meaningful results can still be achieved when these limitations are properly considered or mitigated. An increased adoption of more process-aware information systems would certainly be beneficial for process mining projects, as these can provide the required data directly or will at least do a better job at storing the required data (i.e., the ideal data from Table 4.2).

Table 4.2 The ideal data and the minimal data requirements to get high-quality results

	Ideal	Minimum requirements
Activity events	(Pre)defined events that relate to the activities executed in the process	Enough secondary data to reconstruct the events that relate to the activities executed in the process (i.e., reverse engineering)
Data events	Data related to the decision rationale of, and the source data used by, the process actors when determining the process variant to follow. This includes all data related to the specific context and the defining characteristics of each case	All documented data that was used by the process actors when determining the process variant to follow. So, all available data related to the specific context and the defining characteristics of each case. A process and decision model can be discovered if relevant data is available, but otherwise it can only be a process model
Resource events	(Pre)defined events that relate to the availability, usage and authorization of resources during executed in the process	Enough secondary data to reconstruct the events that relate to the availability, usage and authorization of resources during executed in the process (i.e., reverse engineering)
Timestamps	Timestamps for each activity event and data event, which represent the exact time that the corresponding real-life activity was performed or that the corresponding data element (e.g., lab results) became available to the process actors	A relative order of the activity and data events that represents the order in which the corresponding real-life activities were performed and the corresponding data elements (e.g., lab results) became available to the process actors
Number of cases	Representative set of cases during a period in which no seriously disruptive changes to the process occurred	

4.3.2 Data Preprocessing

The use of a certain type of database management system (DMBS) (e.g., a relational DBMS) imposes specific structural limitations on how data is stored in the database (e.g., data attributes must be single-valued in a relational DBMS). These limitations should not hinder the subsequent steps of the proposed method, and therefore, a conceptual model should to be constructed that makes abstraction of any structural limitations of the original database and other implementation-related aspects (Fig. 4.3).

Aside from database limitations, a typical difficulty of a method such as this one is that much of the data is stored as plain text in the database. This data cannot be used without introducing some additional structure. Text mining and Natural Language Processing [172] techniques can be used to transform the plain text to more structured data, for example TiMBL [173]. Of course, different techniques can be applied without changing the proposed method.

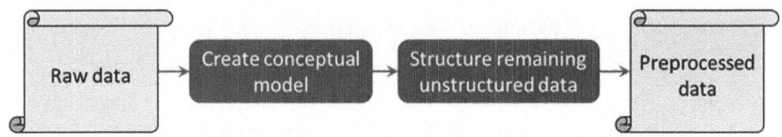

Fig. 4.3 The intermediate activities to go from the raw data to preprocessed data

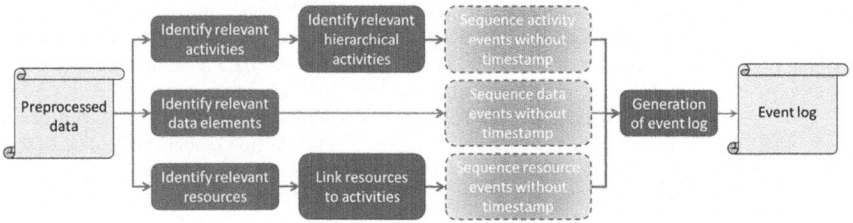

Fig. 4.4 The intermediate activities to go from the preprocessed data to an event log

4.3.3 Log Preparation

In this step, the traces of an event log describing the data need to be reconstructed (Fig. 4.4). This means walking through the data of each historic execution of the process, as structured by the conceptual model, and identifying the relevant activity, data and resource events.

The hierarchical extension of DeciClare allows activities to be grouped as higher-level activities, which in turn can be grouped as even higher-level activities. For example, the activities of 'Request an echo', 'Request a CT' and 'Request an MRI' can be grouped in an activity 'Request a scan', which in turn can be grouped with 'Request lab test' as the activity 'Request diagnostic test'. An activity can also be part of multiple higher-level activities. The definition of higher-level activities will often require some help from a domain expert to ensure domain validity.

We also included three optional intermediate activities in Fig. 4.4 (denoted transparently and with dashed lines). These are not needed when the minimal requirements from Table 4.2 are met. However as noted in Subsect. 4.3.1, this is not always possible in real-life projects. Often there will be some missing events or timestamps in the dataset. These optional intermediate activities facilitate the resolution or mitigation of such data quality issues as much as possible.

4.3.4 Mining a Process and Decision Model

Process mining tools can use the event log composed in the previous steps as input for the discovery of process models (Fig. 4.5). Process mining techniques that create imperative process models often resort to the use of slice and dice, variance-based

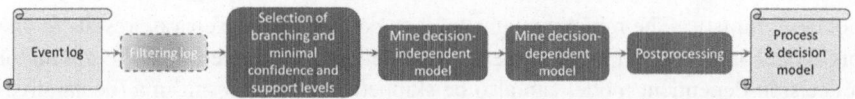

Fig. 4.5 The intermediate activities to go from the event log to an integrated process and decision model

filtering (e.g., clustering) or compliance-based filtering to reduce the complexity of a given event log [34, 35, 160]. For process mining techniques that create declarative process models this is not a necessity, as these can handle more of the complexity, but can also optionally be used to focus on a specific part of the dataset.

While the other activities can be performed mostly automatically, the selection of the maximal branching level and minimal confidence and support levels (see Table 12 for definitions) is more of a judgement call. The minimal confidence and support levels are directly linked to the data quality. These parameters can be used to control the level of detail and complexity of the resulting models in order to prevent overfitting and manage the impact of noise in the event log. Therefore, the consultant responsible for the project should choose good initial values for these parameters. Generally, we would advise to start with a confidence level of 100% (or very close to it) and a minimal support level that corresponds to tens or even hundreds of traces (i.e., 0.1%–2% for a log of 10.000 traces). This will result in a model describing behavior that is never violated in any trace and is reasonably frequently occurring. These levels can be tuned in later iterations based on the results of the evaluation described in the next subsection. If the resulting model contains too many decision-dependent constraints and/or overfitted decision logic, then a step-by-step increase of the minimal support level could improve the results. On the other hand, decreasing the minimal support level is a better course of action when insufficient decision logic was found. The minimal confidence level can also be gradually lowered to counteract the noise in the dataset (i.e., real behavior is not found due to data quality issues or just extreme outliers). A minimal confidence level lower than 100% will allow the mined constraints to be violated by some of the traces in the event log if enough other traces confirm the corresponding behavior pattern. Although DeciClareMiner can mine constraints with lower-than-100% confidence, it can result in inconsistent models [174] and tools to resolve this [175] are not yet available for DeciClare. This means that it can be useful to mine constraints lower-than-100% confidence when the goal is to explain some specific behavior or to expose some pieces of knowledge for human understanding. However, if the goal is to use the mined model as input for a business process engine of a process-aware information system, then constraints lower-than-100% confidence should only be considered after extensive verification. The maximal branching level should preferably be chosen after consulting domain experts and/or process actors. A branching level of one is often the best starting value. Whenever possible, hierarchical activities should be used as they are more computationally efficient and could eliminate the need for higher branching levels.

The second phase of DeciClareMiner, the search for decision-dependent rules, can be executed multiple times with the same parameter settings, as this phase is not deterministic. The miner contains tools to combine these separate results to one big model at the end. If no data events were defined in the event log, the mining of a decision-dependent model can also be skipped. This will result in a (declarative) process model without any data-related decision logic.

Postprocessing is applied automatically to the raw output of DeciClareMiner. This eliminates equivalent decision rules (i.e., combinations of data values that uniquely identify the same cases) and returns a much smaller model with the given minimal support and confidence levels. However, it is not necessarily true that when two decision rules are equivalent in a given event log, that this is also true in the corresponding real-life process. It can be impossible to distinguish between a real-life decision rule and other decision rules that identify the same set of cases due to the incompleteness of the log (i.e., not every possible case occurring). For example, consider the constraint that at least one NMR will be taken. This could apply to patients with a red color code and a remark that mentions the neck, but the same patients might also be identified uniquely with a red color code and the remark that mentions sweatiness (just because this limited set of patients happened to have both).

4.3.5   Evaluation

After each mining step, the correctness of the reconstructed event log and the mined DeciClare-model needs to be evaluated by a domain expert (see Fig. 4.2). Verifying the correctness of the reconstructed event log is the first priority, as it is the input for the mining techniques. Random sampling can be used to select a set of reconstructed traces that will be manually reviewed by domain experts, preferably side-by-side to the original data so that the experts get the full context. This should be repeated until all following stopping criteria are reached:

1. There should be no discrepancies between the original timeline and the reconstructed sequence of activities of the simulated patients (i.e., in the correct order or at least in a realistic order when the original data does not specify an exact time).
2. The available contextual data should be contained by the reconstructed data events. Of course, The focus here is on the essential contextual data that is relevant to the decision-making of process actors.
3. All data events of the simulated patients should be based on data that was actually available at that time in the process (i.e., no data events using data that was added in retrospect or at an unknown time).

When the reconstructed event log is deemed satisfactory, the evaluation of the mined models can begin. The mined process and decision models are difficult to review directly because there is often nothing tangible to compare them with (i.e., tacit knowledge). The understandability issues associated with declarative process models [36] and the typical size of these models also make it infeasible to go over them one-by-one. The type of evaluation needed also depends on the specific use case that the organization has in mind for the mined model.

In general, we would advise the adoption of a similar approach to [176, 177], which uses the visual simulation capabilities of Alloy Analyzer to evaluate a conceptual model, for the simultaneous evaluation of a reconstructed event log and the corresponding mined model. The DeciClareEngine (see 5.1) and its 'Log Replay'-module (Fig. 4.6) can replace Alloy Analyzer to demonstrate what the mined process model knows about what can, must and cannot happen during the execution of specific traces. It can show what activities have been executed at each stage during the replay of a trace (top), the corresponding data events (middle) and the activities that can be executed next according to the mined process model (bottom). The user can view the reasons why a certain activity must/cannot be executed as well as any future restrictions that might apply (in the form of constraints) at any time by clicking on the 'Explanation'-, 'Relevant Model'- and 'Current Restrictions'-buttons. Domain experts can be asked to give feedback during the replay of a random sample of reconstructed traces. Before the execution of each activity, the questions from Table 4.3 can be asked. The answers gauge the correctness of the reconstructed event log (i.e., 1, 2 and 3) and mined model (i.e., 4 and 5) as well as the value of the model to the managers and physicians (i.e., 6).

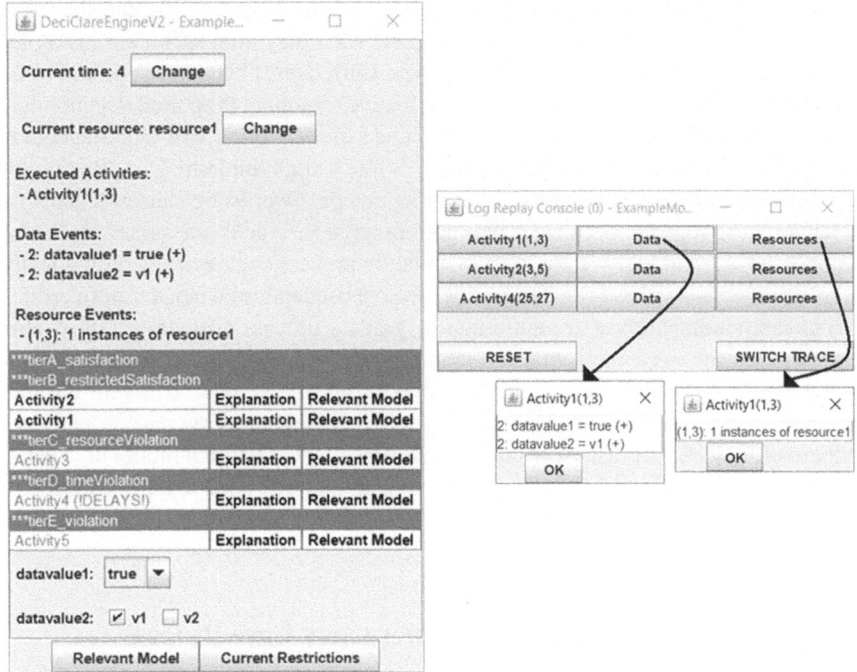

Fig. 4.6 The interface of the DeciClareEngine model simulator (left) and the 'Log Replay'-module for DeciClareEngine (right)

Table 4.3 The questions for the domain experts and the underlying purpose behind each of them for the evaluation

	Question	Purpose
1	Based on the data, are there any activities that might be missing at this point?	*Identify missing activities*
2	Is the order of activities how you would expect based on the data?	*Identify activity reconstruction mistakes*
3	Do the data events generated so far correspond to the data available at this point?	*Identify data reconstruction mistakes*
4	Does the model allow activities to be executed next that should not be allowed?	*Detecting underfit in model*
5	Does the model prohibit activities to be executed next that should be allowed?	*Detecting overfit in model*
6	Does the decision logic for why certain activities are allowed/prohibited reflect real decision-making processes?	*Measuring knowledge extraction of model*

Ideally, the model fit should be perfect. However, this is not realistic for loosely framed knowledge-intensive processes. The main obstacles are the data quality and completeness of the event log. On the one hand, data of insufficient quality can hide acceptable behavior and introduce wrong behavior in models [178]. On the other hand, event logs are almost always incomplete (i.e., they do not contain examples of all acceptable behavior) [179]. Thus, some (infrequent) behavior is bound to be missing in the mined models, even when inductive reasoning is applied to generalize the observed behavior. The result is that mined models often will simultaneously contain some over- and underfitting pieces. While a slight underfit is not that big of a problem for process automation, overfitting can be. Overfitting causes acceptable behavior to be rejected because it was not observed in exactly the same way in the reconstructed event log. We envision that mature process engines will automatically relax or prune away these overfitting rules (i.e., self-adaption) when a user overrules the model, similar to how it would handle gradual process evaluation [180]. This also reduces the need for a full validation of the mined model as it will be validated gradually by the users, with each overfitting rule serving as a warning that the deviating behavior is not typical. Of course, this is not a free pass to purposefully overfit models. It just means that when searching the optimal model fit, a small overfit is manageable and perhaps preferred to an underfit. This feature is currently in development for DeciClareEngine.

4.4   Method Application: The Emergency Care Process

This section provides a brief description of the application of the method presented in the previous section. The practical problem and organizational context that has been tackled is the discovery of an integrated process and decision model of the emergency care process that takes place in the emergency medicine department of a private hospital with 542 beds[1]. Data about the registration, diagnosis and treatment of patients over a span of just under two years is available in their Electronic Health Record (EHR) system. Most of this data is plain text (in Dutch), which is a typical obstacle for process and decision discovery [181]. The role of consultant was performed by the first author as is typical in ADR.

Discovery methods are used as a tool to achieve specific goals in an organization. This method application contained two of the most important use cases for model discovery of loosely framed knowledge-intensive processes in general: a model for operational process automation and a model to extract tacit knowledge related to operational decision-making.

For the first use case, the discovered model should enable operational process automation by serving as the foundation for a context- and process-aware information system [182]. Such a system can support the process actors by enforcing the model (see 5.1) and by providing context-aware recommendations on what to do next (see 5.2). While the former can prevent medical errors, the latter can offer guidance and help optimize the process. The primary goal of the method application was to create a model that facilitates the transition from a process-unaware information system to a context- and process aware information system without disrupting the current working habits. A review of whether every patient in the dataset was handled correctly according to the current medical guidelines was outside the scope of the project, therefore, we assumed that all patients in the dataset were handled correctly. This meant that the goal for the resulting model was to incapsulate the observed behavior from the reconstructed event log and also allow unobserved behavior that follows similar logic, while at the same time restricting other unobserved behavior as much as possible.

Medical personnel typically leverage their knowledge and experience when deciding on how to deal with a specific patient. This knowledge can apply to all patients (e.g., registration always first) or to a specific subset of patients based on the characteristics of the patient and other context variables (e.g., if shoulder pain and sweaty, then take echo of the heart). This kind of knowledge is typically not explicitly available anywhere, but rather contained in the minds of the physicians. The second use case consists of transforming such tacit knowledge into explicit knowledge, which can be used in many ways: it can be discussed amongst physicians to promote transparency and ensure uniformity, used to train new physicians and nurses, to improve resource planning (e.g., can reserve some slots for patients that will need an MRI based on their contexts, even though it has not been formally requested yet), etc. Therefore, the goal for the resulting model was to discover useful and realistic medical knowledge.

---

[1] AZ Maria Middelares hospital, Ghent, Belgium - https://www.mariamiddelares.be/

4.4.1   Extraction

The hospital provided us with an export of six database tables from their internally developed EHR system spanning the period from 31/12/2015 until 22/09/2017. The data was exported from the original relational DBMS in the form of anonymized CSV-files. The minimum requirements from Table 4.2 were not satisfied because of some missing timestamps and a lack of data related to the availability, usage and authorization of the resources during the execution of the process.

4.4.2   Data Preprocessing

Figure 4.7 presents the conceptual model that was reconstructed from the raw EHR data. A care episode represents a single admittance of a patient that can end with a discharge or a transfer to another department. The plain text data fields were structured by transforming them each to a set of keywords.

4.4.3   Log Preparation

Next, we reconstructed the chronology and created a trace for each care episode. The reconstruction of the activity events is illustrated with an example in Fig. 4.8. The activity events are shown in blue with the elapsed time between brackets (corresponding data events are omitted). The green arrows link the activity events with the data on which they are based. The relevant data values are transformed to data events

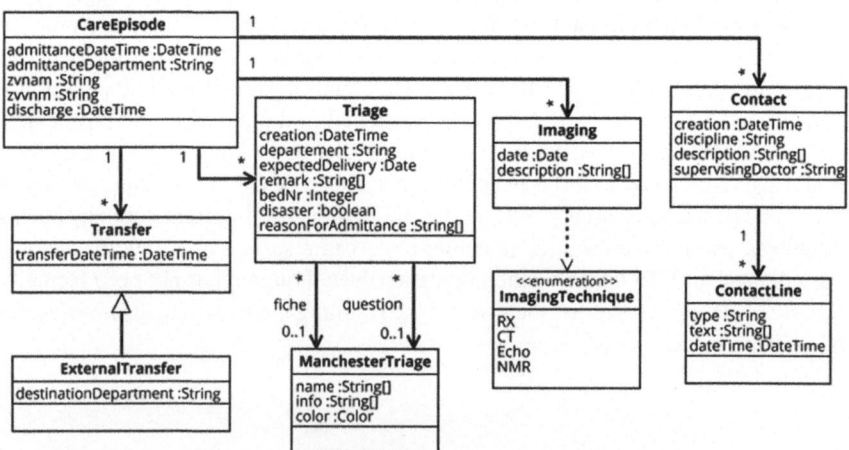

Fig. 4.7 UML class diagram of the conceptual model for the preprocessed data

Table 4.4 Additional statistics on the event log

	Total of all traces	Minimum per trace	Maximum per trace	Average per trace	Median per trace
Duration (hours)	133686	0.067	22.3	3.2	2.9
#Activity events	625682	3	128	15	17
#Data events	1350331	2	166	32.4	32

in the trace. The most interesting data to reconstruct the decision logic of the process is stored in the plain text attributes (e.g., the attribute 'text' in the ContactLine-class), which have been preprocessed to multisets of keywords as described in Subsect. 4.3.2. For each of those attributes, the keywords were transformed to categorical data events (e.g., 'Description of Medical history' = 'foot'). Practically, we used the XES-format for the event log and used a custom extension to include general data events (i.e., adds data events with a timestamp that do not need to be directly linked to an activity event).

Several iterations were needed to create a satisfactory event log. Yet, the need for these iterations only can come up during later steps because a domain expert must make this assessment. It would be possible to add an intermediate evaluation of the constructed event log at the end of this step, depending on the urgency of the project and the availability of the domain expert. However, the next step (mining) is automated anyway. Therefore, we decided against adding the extra evaluation step. We just used the created event log to mine a model and had the domain expert evaluate the event log and mined model simultaneously during the normal evaluation step. The first iterations of the event log creation focused on the identification and granularity of activities and data elements, while the sequencing of activities with missing timestamps (i.e., imaging activities and lab tests) also required multiple iterations. Each iteration incrementally improved the event log to better reflect reality. The resulting event log contains 41657 traces using 116 unique activities and 951 unique data values. Some additional statistics about the log are presented in Table 4.4.

4.4.4   Mining a Process and Decision Model

DeciClareMiner was executed on an Intel Xeon Gold 6140 with the emergency care event log from Subsect. 4.4.3 and several different parameter settings as input. The maximal branching level was set at 1 (i.e., no branching). Some smaller scale experiments with higher branching levels showed a significant increase in model size with little added value. The definition of 15 hierarchical activities also reduced the need for higher branching levels. We started with a minimal confidence level of 100% (i.e., only never-violated behavior was mined) and a minimal support level of 10%

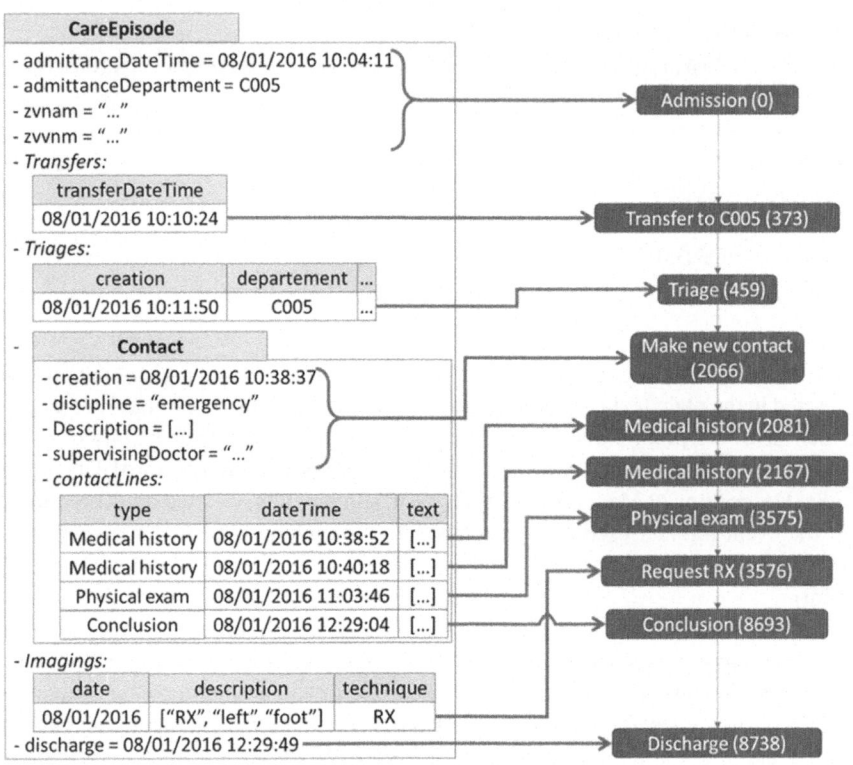

Fig. 4.8 An example of how the internal representation (preprocessed data) is transformed to a trace

(i.e., only behavior that was observed in minimally 4166 of 41657 traces). These two values were iteratively adjusted to improve the quality of the results. Minimal support levels were relaxed from 10% to 5%, 2%, 1%, 0.24%, 0.048%, 0.024%, 0.012% and 0.007%. These values were not chosen randomly, but rather based on the minimal number of observations we wanted for the discovered behavior patterns (e.g., 0.007% corresponds to a minimum of three observations). In the context of the second use case, we also mined models with minimal confidence levels of 98%, 97.5%, 96.67%, 95% and 90% in order to also find knowledge patterns that are otherwise hidden due to noise in the data. The results[2] consist of a post-processed model for the evaluation of the first use case and the raw model used for the evaluation of the second use case.

---

[2] https://github.com/stevmert/discoveryMethod

4.4.5   Evaluation

We used DeciClareEngine and its 'Log Replay'-module for the evaluation of the model of the emergency care process. We also created an additional module to visualize the original data plain text of the EHR side-by-side with the trace and its keyword representations of those texts to facilitate the evaluation of the reconstructed event log. The 'Log Replay'-module and the new custom module have an interface that gives an overview of the activities of the trace on the left and 'Data'-buttons on the right (left side of Fig. 4.9). Clicking on one of the activities will set the state of the engine to just after the execution of that activity, while the original EHR data can be opened by clicking on the 'Data'-button next to each activity (right side of Fig. 4.9). This was used to replay the care episodes of many patients for the domain expert. He was asked the questions from Table 4.3 before and after each activity in a replayed trace. Hence, it was an evaluation using sampling and validation of the model in the context of specific patients, and not on a per constraint basis. The evaluation helped identify several issues with the reconstructed event log as well as with the mined models. These issues were handled during subsequent iterations of the method. This was repeated until a satisfactory result was reached (taking into account the data quality of the available dataset).

The result of the first use case, the discovery of a model for operational process automation, is an operational model of the emergency care process that takes place in the emergency medicine department of the AZ Maria Middelares hospital in Belgium. The model contains 28162 decision-independent and 6283 decision-dependent constraints. The minimal confidence level setting of 100% and the application of induction by the mining technique resulted in a model that was sufficiently flexible and general to serve as input for a business process engine (e.g., DeciClareEngine) of a context- and process-aware information system. Figure 4.10 presents a simplification of the decision-independent constraints of the model using the Declare visual syntax [22]. It shows only the activities done by emergency physicians (so no specialist activities), combines the external transfers that do not have a specific relation constraint into a generalized activity called 'External transfer (other)', omits chain constraints and omits other constraints with a support lower than 0.25%.

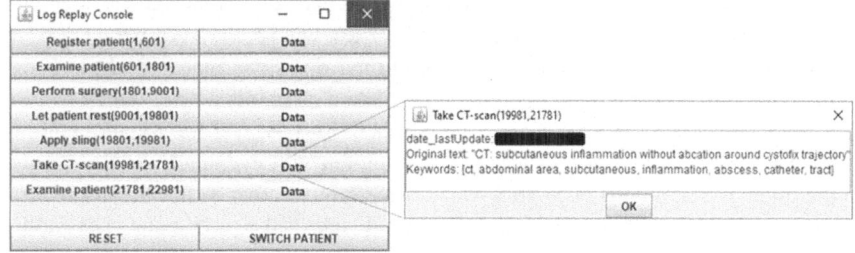

Fig. 4.9 The log replay console that can replay a trace up to every decision point and display the original EHR data for the simulated patient

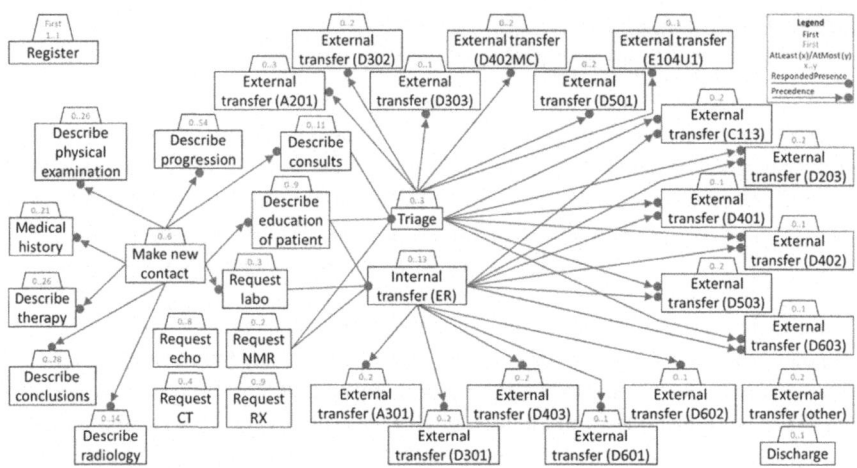

Fig. 4.10 Simplified Declare representation of the mined process model

The model created for the first use case provides a rare peek into the daily operation of an emergency medicine department. The model reveals the patterns and the specific contexts that some of the patterns apply to. The broad outlines of the model were not surprising to any of the process actors, as they already had an implicit idea of the general way things are done at the department, but the model makes them explicit so that it becomes accessible to outsiders (e.g., management, emergency physicians in training, patients, etc.). However, from the point of view of knowledge extraction things get more interesting when diving deeper into a model. The model from the first use case is limited to behavior that is not violated in any of the observations in the event log in order to be suited for operational use. This means that even the slightest inaccuracy of the source data, due to either forgetfulness or incompetence, will prevent the discovery of certain valid behavior and decision patterns no matter its frequency of occurrence.

The knowledge currently captured by a model mined with DeciClareMiner consists of two main components: the functional and control-flow perspectives describing the occurrence and sequencing rules concerning the activities and the decision logic that determines the context in which each occurrence and sequencing rule applies. The second use case focusses on the knowledge that was extracted from the reconstructed event log about the operational decisions made by the process actors. This refers to the data contexts that make constraints active, which in turn can require or block the execution of certain activities (e.g., if the triage mentions an overdose and respiratory issues, then the patient will eventually be transferred to the intensive care unit). The goal was to ascertain whether or not the discovered decision logic matched the tacit medical knowledge of the physicians. The model did not need to be executable for this use case. Therefore, it combined the results of the first use case with additional mining results with minimal confidence levels lower than 100%.

We used an evaluation consisting of two parts for this second use case. The same setup as for the first use case was used in the first part because this allowed for an efficient validation of the reconstruction of the event log as well as showed some of the activation decisions in a real context. The second part entailed a direct evaluation of the activation decisions of selected constraints. The disjunct pieces of decision logic were listed for each of the constraints, which facilitated a Likert-scale scoring by domain experts based on (medical) correctness of each activating data context. The domain expert was subsequently asked to evaluate some of the discovered decision criteria for when certain activities need to be executed. For example, if the patient received a green color code during the triage and the medical discipline of the care episode is ophthalmology, then the patient would eventually be discharged. Note that this type of rules (i.e., positive) are the most interesting but also the most difficult to discover. A lot of decision logic related to negative rules was also discovered, but this is less interesting due to those rules being less helpful and typically common sense (e.g., a patient with dementia should never be transferred to Neonatology). The domain expert evaluated 208 discovered decision criteria for when the following activities are executed at least once: Patient Discharge, Request CT, Request RX, Transfer to Pediatrics, Transfer to Oncology/Nephrology, Transfer to Cardiology and Transfer to Geriatrics. Each disjunct part of the discovered decision logic was listed and subsequently scored on a Likert-scale ranging from medical nonsense to realistic decision logic. The results are summarized in Fig. 4.11. We also included the results of an intermediate version of this evaluation to show the evolution after several iterations of the proposed method.

The results show that around 53% of the decision criteria were evaluated as real-istic in the final evaluation, although some small nuances were often missing. This highlights the potential value of the proposed method to automatically transform tacit

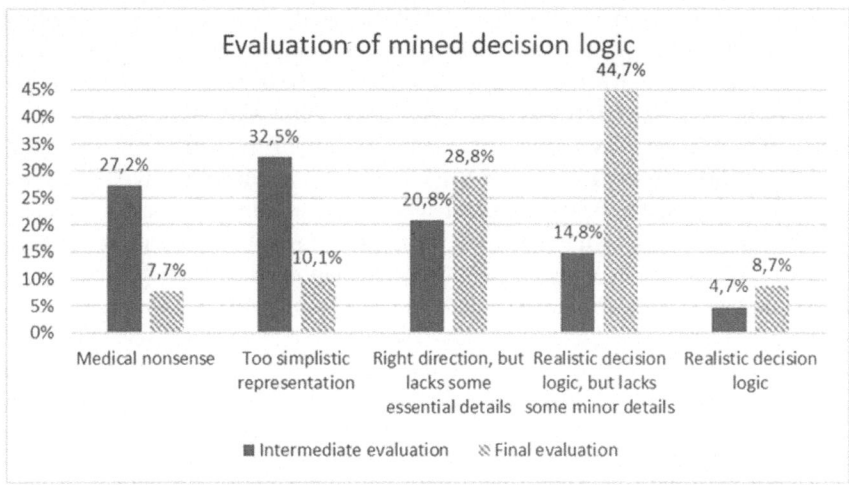

Fig. 4.11 The results of the evaluations of the mined decision logic by the domain expert

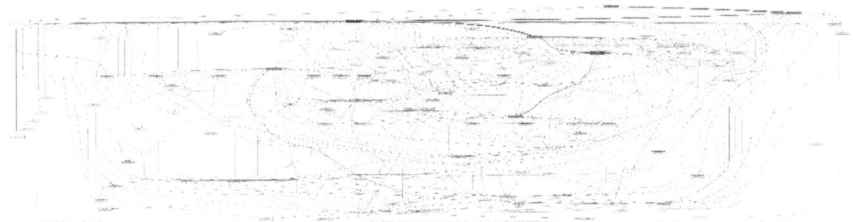

Fig. 4.12 The imperative process model as generated by the Disco-tool

to explicit knowledge in healthcare, and more generally, for all sorts of loosely framed knowledge-intensive processes. The improvements over the intermediate evaluation demonstrate the need for multiple iterations. The model used in the intermediate evaluation contained much more nonsense, primarily due to the use of lower minimal support levels during the mining step. Much of this nonsense was filtered out of the model by increasing the minimal support level.

4.4.6 Discussion

The work is based on the premise that imperative modeling techniques are not suitable for loosely framed processes, which includes many healthcare processes. Figure 4.12 presents an imperative process model mined from the same event log created in this section[3]. The model was created by the Disco-tool[4], which was also used to mine a model for an emergency medicine department in Rojas et al. [160]. It contains all activities but ignores the data events (as this feature is not supported by the tool) and shows just the 1.1% most frequently travelled paths. This is a good example of how traditional process discovery techniques would represent the emergency care process of the AZ Maria Middelares hospital. Despite the omission of data events and 90.1% of the less frequently travelled paths, the result is still an unreadable model that is often referred to as a spaghetti model [10, 160]. This is caused by the 28980 unique variations in the log (out of 41657 patients), as identified by Disco when only considering the activity events, of which the most frequent variation occurs just 686 times (1.65%). An imperatively process discovery tool either interconnects almost every activity to include each of these variations (i.e., unreadable spaghetti model) or filters out all complexity to only leave some sort of generalized happy path (i.e., does not reflect reality). This is a typical problem when modeling healthcare processes imperatively that results in poor usability of the resulting models [156, 183]. Rojas et al. worked around this by asking domain experts to manually

---

[3] A version of the image in the highest export resolution available in Disco is available at https://git hub.com/stevmert/discoveryMethod/

[4] https://fluxicon.com/disco/

define subsets of activities that are expected to be part of smaller and more manageable subprocesses, while Duma and Aringhieri [156] resort to making significant assumptions and simplifications. Declarative modeling languages are better suited to these processes [16], because they actually extract the logical rules that define the connections between activities instead of just enumerating the most frequently encountered connections like imperative techniques do. The DeciClare language used in our method caters specifically to loosely framed knowledge-intensive healthcare processes with its integrated data perspective, which enables even more fine-grained knowledge to be extracted from the data.

The process and decision model created during the application of the proposed method certainly revealed some useful insight into the emergency care process of the AZ Maria Middelares hospital. Despite the basic (rather than advanced) data analysis and other limitations, it managed to transform a lot of tacit knowledge into valuable and explicit knowledge. Of course, much of the discovered knowledge was already known to the experienced physicians in the department, but now it is also readily available to less experienced physicians and other stakeholders that want to gain insight into the operation of an emergency medicine department. Having explicit rules for the occurrence and sequencing of activities and the corresponding decision logic available enables deeper analysis and optimization of the working habits of the emergency physicians. Both use cases showed the potential of the proposed method to make previously tacit knowledge explicitly available for all stakeholders, for both operational and decision-making purposes. Process and decision models, like the one mined in this chapter, have the potential to unlock a new tier of applications further along the line. For example:

- An explicit justification as to why certain activities are performed in specific cases and others are not.
- The decision logic of treatments in the model can be compared to the available clinical guidelines. Do the physicians follow the guidelines? If not, what are the characteristic and decision criteria of the cases in which they diverge from the guidelines? Are these justifiable?
- The decision logic of different physicians can be compared. Do the physicians treat similar patients similarly? What are the differences? Can adjustments be made to make the service level more uniform?
- The knowledge contained by models will make simulations much more realistic and flexible. For example, how would a department address an increase in a group of pathologies by 5%? Would this create new bottlenecks? Can these be eliminated by changing, if possible, some decision criteria?
- The knowledge made explicit by the mined models can be used to bring interns more quickly up to speed or even to educate future nurses/physicians as part of their medical training.
- The mined models can be used for evidence farming [147]. This is the practice of posteriori analysis of clinical data to find new insights without setting up case-control studies. Evidence farming can be used as an alternative or, even better, as a supplement to evidence-based medicine.

Throughout the application of the developed method, we encountered several typical limitations of process discovery projects. Different types of noise in the data that was used to create the model are the primary limitation. This is real-life data that was recorded without this sort of applications in mind, so it would be unrealistic to expect perfect data. The data quality framework of Vanbrabant et al. classifies 14 data quality problems typical to electronic healthcare records of emergency departments in several (sub)categories: missing data, dependency violations, incorrect attribute values and data that is not wrong but not directly usable [184]. All 14 data quality problems were encountered at one point or another during this project. In terms of the forms of noise defined by van der Spoel et al., we encountered the following [185]:

- Sequence noise: errors in, or uncertainty about, the order of events in an event trace.

In this project we did not have an exact timestamp of the radiology and lab activities. So, a workaround was devised that is by no means perfect. Additionally, the timestamps that we did have are those of when the physicians or nurses describe activities in the EHR, but this does not necessarily reflect the timing and order of the actual activities performed. Some physicians prefer to update the EHR of a patient for several activities simultaneously. Consequently, the preservation of the sequence information is dependent on whether physicians describe those activities in the same order as they performed them (which was generally the case). Although there is no way to fully resolve this issue, aside from a whole new system to record the data, we did use names for the activities that correctly reflect the data that we had. Many activities were named like 'Describe …' or 'Request …' to signify that we cannot make a statement about when the actual activity occurred, just when the description or request was made.

- Duration noise: noise arising from missing or wrong timestamps for activities and variable duration between activities.

The issues described for sequence noise also apply here. We only had timestamps of when an update was saved to the EHR. Hence, there was no timestamp of the actual activity or even a duration. We gave every activity an arbitrary duration of two seconds for practical reasons, but this does not reflect reality.

- Human noise: noise from human errors such as activities in a care path which were the result of a wrong or faulty diagnosis or from a faulty execution of a treatment or procedure.

When writing in the EHR, physicians and nurses will unavoidably make mistakes: typos, missing text, missing activity descriptions, activity descriptions entered in the incorrectly activity text field… But even correct description of activities can cause problems as a different jargon will make it more difficult to detect patterns. We preprocessed the plain text data to resolve the more frequent typos and used a list of synonyms and generalizations to deal with the use of different jargons. However, these solutions are not exhaustive, and thus, could still be improved. The release of an official dictionary and thesaurus of medical jargon in the Dutch language would be a big step in the right direction.

Two other general limitations related to data completeness typical for process mining projects also applies to this project. Firstly, process mining starts with an assumption of event log completeness [161]. This means that we assume that every possible trace variation (i.e., type of patient, diagnosis, complication, treatment, etc.) that can occur also occurred in the event log. Of course, this is not realistic as each event log contains just a subset of these variations. The result is that the process models will generally overfit the event log (i.e., it was never observed that a patient needed more than four CT-scans, so the model says this cannot occur, while there might be infrequent cases for which this could be possible). This can be mitigated during the project by fiddling with the minimal support level for the mining step and after the project by slowly gathering more and more data. The second general limitation relates to the completeness of the context data. Decision mining works best when all the data used by the process actors during the execution of the process is available in the event log. However, due to privacy concerns this is difficult to achieve, especially in healthcare. In our case, we did not get access to several general patient attributes (e.g., age and gender) as well as to any information about the medical history of the patients. Of course, this severely limits what can be discovered. And finally, we encountered the following event log imperfection patterns [178]: form-based event capture, unanchored events, scattered events, elusive cases and polluted labels.

The issues described above lead to a loss of accuracy in the resulting process and decision model. Some knowledge is lost, while other knowledge that was discovered does not correctly reflect reality. Furthermore, the model only considers the emergency medicine department of one hospital. The generalizability of the model is therefore low. Every hospital and/or department has their own capabilities, limitations and way of doing things.

During this case study, several ideas and opportunities came up to increase the success rate of similar projects in the future at the emergency medicine department of AZMM. The benefits of storing additional process-related information became more concrete, which further increases the willingness to make changes to the current situation. Some ideas entail changes to the underlying information system. For example, storing more timestamps concerning radiology and lab activities (i.e., time of request, time of execution, time when the results were made available, time when the physician looks at the results…). While other ideas involve to more radical changes to the way that the medical personnel go about their business. A medical scribe was made available during a test period to relief the physicians of most of the writing activities in the EHR and at the same time to make the input more uniform. An expansion of the current capabilities to generate default texts based on shortcuts is also under consideration, possibly in combination with all options/answers so that the physician just needs to remove what is not applicable instead of having to type it. An even more ambitious idea of adding some sort of spelling correction to interface of the EHR was also discussed. All this extra structure in the textual input of the EHR will result in more precise data in the future, and consequently, more precise process models.

Table 4.5 A summary of the lessons learned for data scientists

	Lesson	Description
1	*Start with a specific goal in mind*	It is important to define and discuss the goal(s) of the discovery project beforehand with the managers and physicians. The specific goals can have a significant impact on several steps of the method application. In this work, we described two use cases with different goals that required different minimal confidence and support levels and evaluation. Other interesting use cases could focus on the physicians providing the treatment. For example, discovering a model that only includes patients that were treated by the more experienced physicians or a model per physician to compare them internally. Each of these use cases would require different implementations of the selection of data extracted from the information system and/or the event log filtering steps
2	*The available data, data selection and data quality remain crucial*	The process and decision discovery method is an important part of a discovery project. Yet, it is the available process data that will determine whether the project goals are achievable, even when everything else is done perfectly. The method will not produce any useful results without the right data of sufficiently high quality. This is essentially the 'garbage in, garbage out'-principle. Perfect data does not exist in real-life projects, so it is important to be aware of the imperfections and, where possible, try to mitigate them. Being aware of the data issues is also important to prevent wrong conclusions from being drawn from the results Perhaps the most important role here is played by the domain expert(s) supporting the data scientists. Good domain experts have experiences on the work floor and are preferably still active there. As a data scientist, it is essential to thoroughly explain what you need and what the eventual goals are to the domain experts. If they fully understand those, they can anticipate your needs and point you in the right direction. Also involve them as much as possible in the data selection and quality review. They can give valuable insight into what is being inputted into the system and how trustworthy this data is
		In our method application, we had to deal with multiple data problems such as data not being registered, not having access to certain useful data (e.g., no patient age or gender due to patient privacy regulations), pruning out unrelated or low quality data attributes and managing different types of noise. Therefore, we performed a critical review of the available data with together with people from different levels of the organization: After a thorough discussion of the purpose of the discovery method, we defined the project with the head of the emergency department. This included a review of the information system as used on the work floor to get a good feel for what is being recorded and the subsequent opportunities for the potential goals of the project. This provided the foundation for the data selection, although at this point still in terms of data inputs of the information system The IT-department provided a mapping of the data inputs in the information system to the model of the extracted data. This revealed the extent to which the requested data was scattered across multiple databases and some other problems for which we had to devise mitigation strategies The physicians were asked to explain how they made use of certain data input fields in the information system. This uncovered some misalignments between how the intended usage by the IT-department and the actual usage by the physicians, as well as some creative use to get around certain limitations. Based on this information, we could prune out certain low-quality data attributes and implement several data quality improvement steps Together with the head of the emergency department, who was also our domain expert, we subsequently ran through many process instances during the evaluation step to review both the quality of the data and of the model based on that data. This exposed additional data issues, like registered data that was not provided to us or misinterpreted data. Most of these issues could be solved during a subsequent iteration of the method The remaining data and quality issues were documented during the method application and linked to certain parts of the discovered model to make the eventual users of the model aware of its weaknesses

(continued)

Table 4.5 (continued)

	Lesson	Description
3	*Favor hierarchical activities over branching*	The underlying process logic often involves more than the minimal number of activities linked to a certain declarative rule. Increasing the branching level will allow the miner to discover more of this logic. However, the percentage of spurious relationships in the results will likely rise and the added computational effort is very high. When possible, hierarchical activities should be defined to group some lower level activities or even other hierarchical activities. This is a manual step that requires some domain knowledge but could certainly pay dividends later down the line. Mining hierarchical activities is much more computationally efficient and prevents many of the spurious relationships to be discovered. If the domain knowledge is not available to define the hierarchical activities, one can still resort to higher branching levels when the sufficient computational power is available
4	*The identification of data elements is a tough balancing exercise*	A naive approach to the identification of data elements might be 'the more the merrier'. After all, the discovery of decision logic depends on having the necessary data elements in the event log. Yet, the practical reality is that this is a difficult trade-off between potentially uncovering more of the real decision logic versus the general quality of the discovered decision logic and the computational effort. Lower quality data elements might lower the quality of the mined model because they could be incorrectly linked to certain discovered decisions, while they also significantly increase the search space leading to a lot of waste mining time. Therefore, the identification and selection of data elements to use in the event log should be done with much care
		We would advise to start from a small set of potential data element candidates, manually review the quality as much as possible and iteratively increase/refine the data elements throughout the project based on the results of the evaluation step at the end of each iteration
5	*Test multiple parameter combinations in parallel*	The selection of the maximal branching level and minimal confidence and support levels can be a bit of trial and error. It is not wrong to choosing one specific combination of values for these parameters for each iteration, but it can be inefficient. By mining with multiple parameter combination per iteration, comparisons can be made of the results early in the project. The different models can be evaluated in the same evaluation step at the end of each iteration to save some time
		Also, keep in mind that the mining step is not deterministic nor complete. Parameter combinations that range from general (high support) to specific (low support) and strict (high confidence) to more lenient (low confidence) can be chosen so that the more general and strict parameter settings are subsumed by each subsequent parameter setting with less general and more lenient levels. So, all models that are more general and stricter can be merged directly in the other models. In general, all the rules in the discovered models can be combined and new models of each parameter combination can be created by filtering the rules with the specific thresholds. The resulting models will be more complete because the search space directly or indirectly explored in these models will be at least equal to, but almost always bigger than, the search space explored during each of the original mining steps. This means that the additional computational effort required to mine more than one model per iteration for internal comparison is optimally leveraged to increase the quality of all models

The method application described in this section required a substantial amount of manual work. This is typical for process mining projects, and even more so in healthcare settings [122]. The intrinsic complexity of the processes and the characteristic process-unaware information systems are the main culprits here. The long-term goal of the overarching research project and the emergency medicine department involved in the case is therefore, respectively, the development of and transition to a context- and process-aware information system. Such a system should understand the process and store the required data directly (e.g., an event log), which eliminates much of the manual work aside from the evaluation. From a research perspective, the manual work performed in the case confirms the need for such a system and provides a glimpse behind the scenes of a real-life loosely frame knowledge-intensive process. The healthcare organization on the other hand can view the manual work as a necessary investment to gather insight into the process taking place in order to facilitate the transition to a more process-aware information system in the future. But even when an organization is not eying a transition to a more process-aware information system, the amount of manual work can be regarded as an investment. Process mining projects are meant to be part of a BPM lifecycle in an organization [1], which specifically states that it is a cycle that needs to be repeated on a continuous basis. Thus, the manual work performed in the first iteration does not need to be redone each iteration, but rather, can be reused in the following iterations. As a result, the amount of manual work will be much lower in later iterations.

Finally, the proposed method should be regarded as a mere tool for process and decision discovery. With that, we mean that its success will depend heavily on the way it is applied. In Table 4.5, we provide a summary of the lessons we learned during this research and application project. These lessons are geared towards the data scientists who will be responsible for applying the method in future discovery projects. We have already touched upon some of these in the previous sections, but here we take a step back and discuss them on a project level.

4.5   Conclusion and Future Research

This chapter describes the application of ADR to develop a method for process and decision discovery for loosely framed knowledge-intensive healthcare processes, centered around the DeciClareMiner tool. The method describes the steps to proceed from raw data in the IT-system of an organization to a detailed process and decision model of such a process. The use of a declarative process mining technique with integrated decision discovery is novel and requires modified approach compared to existing methods for process mining based on imperative process mining techniques. As part of the ADR-cycle, DeciClareMiner was applied for the first time to a real-life loosely framed knowledge-intensive healthcare process, namely the one that is performed in the emergency medicine department of a private hospital. This process is one of (if not the) most diverse, multi-disciplinary and dynamic processes in a hospital. Consequently, process and decision discovery in this setting is very challenging. Most of the process mining papers in a healthcare setting focus on a limited number of steps, aspects or pathologies (e.g., clinical pathways) to reduce the complexity of the task at hand. In contrast, the scope of this project was set out to be as comprehensive as possible with the available data. All recorded activities performed as part of the process in the emergency medicine department as well as all pathologies were considered from the viewpoint of the functional, control-flow and data perspectives of the process without resorting to filtering or clustering techniques to reduce the complexity.

The 'spaghetti' model that resulted from applying an imperative process mining technique to the data (Fig. 4.12) further strengthens the claim that imperative process modeling is not suitable for this type of processes. The understandability advantages (for human users) of imperative over declarative languages is completely negated by the high flexibility needs of the process and the resulting enumeration of all possible paths. Declarative languages are better suited due to their implicit incorporation of process variations. The combination of this declarative viewpoint and an extensive data perspective enables DeciClare models to capture both the loosely framed and the knowledge-intensive characteristics of the targeted processes. As a result, the discovered DeciClare model of the emergency care process offers a glimpse into the previously tacit knowledge about how patients are diagnosed and treated at the emergency medicine department of the hospital. Transforming this tacit knowledge to explicit knowledge can have many benefits to the department, the hospital and possibly even to the medical field in general (e.g., transparency, analysis, comparison, optimization, education...). The evaluation demonstrates that realistic functional, control-flow and decision logic can be identified with the developed method.

This research contributes to the information systems community by bringing together the state-of-the-art from different fields like computer science, business process management, conceptual modeling, process mining, decision management and knowledge representation to make advancements in the field of medical informatics. Although many advancements have recently been made in process mining research, most of the proposed techniques and methods are either geared towards tightly framed processes or lack support for the knowledge governing the path decisions. We have addressed this research gap for the discovery of loosely framed knowledge-intensive healthcare processes. The proposed method is not merely a theoretical contribution, it is a practical contribution. This was demonstrated by the application of the method to a real-life example process, which both shows it feasibility and its potential. Data scientists can use this as a template to create similar models in other healthcare organizations. We envision the method and corresponding tools to be integrated into the hospital information systems of the future to allow for the automatic discovery of such models directly. This could become part of the review process that many healthcare organizations already undergo periodically to verify that clinical guidelines and hospital policies are being applied correctly. On the other hand, the model itself enables the use of process engines like DeciClareEngine that offer automatic interpretation of the model and support users while executing the process by providing them with the right pieces of knowledge at the right time. This is a necessary step towards offering real-time process and decision support covering the complete process, as opposed to current generation of clinical decision support systems that only offer support at some very specific decision point(s) (e.g., for the prevention venous thromboembolism [186]).

As future research, we need to make a distinction between the developed method and the practical case through which the method was developed. In the context of the method, we will further refine it by applying it to other healthcare process, while following the recommendations of Martin et al. [187]. We will also verify its general applicability to other loosely framed knowledge-intensive processes by applying it to datasets from other domains. From the perspective of the practical case, a project like this does not really have a definite ending. It will need to be repeated continuously as initiatives to improve the data quality start to bear fruit. The quality of the discovered process and decision model will improve with more and better data, which in turn externalizes more and more real-life medical knowledge. Additionally, we are investigating how the process and decision model can be used to help users during the execution of the process. The process engine used in the evaluation of the discovered model is a first step in this direction, yet the development of a true context- and process-aware information system is still ongoing.

Research Contribution of Chapter 4
A method for declarative process and decision discovery, describing the steps starting from the data extraction up to the discovery of a satisfactory model of a given process

Chapter 5
Operational Support for Loosely Framed Knowledge-Intensive Processes

This chapter consists of two related parts. The first part is the result of EC5 and describes the development of a data-aware BPE that supports the execution of a declarative process model. The second part is the result of the first iteration of EC6 and RC4-6 and describes the evaluation and comparison of forty strategies to generate next-activity recommendations. The combination of these two subcomponents produces a fully operational BPE, which ensures that the process is executed in conformance to a given process model while also providing recommendations that support process actors during the execution of a process instance.

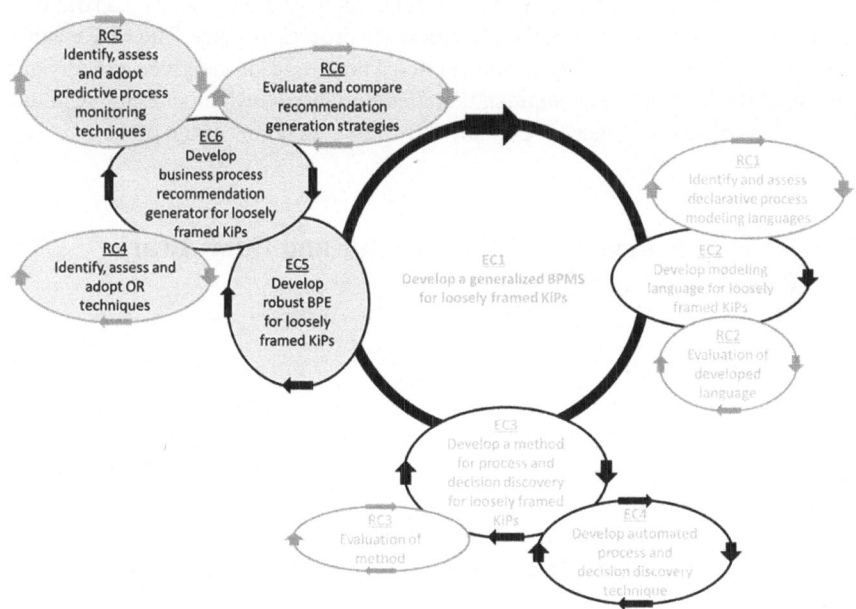

© Springer Nature Switzerland AG 2020
S. Mertens: Enabling Process Management for Loosely Framed
Knowledge-Intensive Processes, LNBIP 409,
https://doi.org/10.1007/978-3-030-66193-9_5

§5.1: Mertens, S., Gailly, F., and Poels, G.: *A Generic Framework for Flexible and Data-Aware Business Process Engines*. In: H. Proper and J. Stirna (eds.) FAISE Workshop at CAiSE'19. LNBIP, vol. 349, pp. 201–213, Springer, Cham (2019).
https://doi.org/10.1007/978-3-030-20948-3_18

§5.2: © 2019 IEEE. Reprinted, with permission, from Mertens, S., Gailly, F., Van Sassenbroeck, D., Poels, G.: *Comparing strategies to generate experience-based clinical process recommendations that leverage similarity to historic data*. In: 2019 IEEE International Conference on Healthcare Informatics (ICHI). IEEE (2019).
https://doi.org/10.1109/ichi.2019.8904693

This chapter consists of two related parts. The Sect. 5.1 describes development of a data-aware BPE that supports the execution of a declarative process model. The resulting BPE, called DeciClareEngine, can execute a given DeciClare model by categorizing every activity according to its availability for execution as the next activity at any time during the execution of a process instance. However, loosely framed KiPs typically have a number of activities that can be executed next, presented as an unsorted set of possible next activities by DeciClareEngine. Hence, it does not always offer much direct guidance to the process actors. The needed guidance can be added by way of a recommendation generator that uses past process instances to rank the available next activities. Section 5.2 provides an implementation of forty strategies to generate next-activity recommendations and describes the evaluation and comparison of these strategies. A recommendation generator based on these implementations is arguably not a part of the BPE-component itself, but rather of the Process Analytics-component of a BPMS (see Sect. 1.1) as an additional layer on top of the BPE. The combination of these two subcomponents provides full operational support to process actors during the execution of a process instance. The BPE ensures that the execution conforms with the explicit knowledge of the given process and decision model, while the recommendation engine offers insight and guidance into the implicit experiences that are contained by past executions of the process.

5.1   A Generic Framework for Flexible and Data-Aware Business Process Engines

5.1.1   Introduction

Loosely framed processes are processes that can be executed in a large, but finite, number of ways with all possible activities known in advance [6, 7, 137]. Example domains are healthcare (e.g., diagnosis and treatment of a patient), legal (e.g., preparing, arguing and pleading a case), helpdesk (e.g., finding a satisfactory solution) and air traffic control (e.g., deciding the priority for the arriving/departing planes). To model loosely framed processes, declarative process modeling languages are the preferred choice due to their implicit support for process flexibility [7, 16, 17, 137]. At the same time, these processes can also be classified as knowledge-intensive

(KiP) [6, 137]: they require knowledge workers (e.g., doctors) to leverage their domain knowledge in search for an appropriate process variation for each case. Therefore, declarative modeling language should also incorporate some form of decision logic, as this allows the domain knowledge to be captured that is essential to the execution of these processes. Declarative process models are often difficult for humans to create and to understand [36]. The innate complexity of the processes themselves is the leading cause, however, the absence of a clear path or flow through the models is a strong second. It is easy to lose sight of the overall process when confronted with a large set of constraints, of which each only applies to specific contexts that can vary widely from one constraint to the next. Moreover, it is hard to capture the tacit knowledge of knowledge workers, accumulated during years of experience, in an explicit process model manually (e.g., through interviews). Process mining techniques can be used to overcome this issue by (semi-)automatically creating models from historic data logs of the process, if available. With a model of the process available, whether it be an original or redesigned version of a manually or automatically created model, the next step is to make sure that future process executions are in conformance with the model. However, due to the aforementioned understandability issues, doing this manually is challenging.

A Business Process Engine (BPE) enables process actors to correctly execute process models by enacting them [188]. A BPE manages the workflow by monitoring and validating the execution, by showing an overview of the partially executed process instance and the restriction that currently apply based on the model, and by notifying the responsible process actors or automated services when needed. The complexity of the models is less of an issue for BPEs, because computers are well equipped for this type of complexity. Although there exist many BPEs for imperative process models, the offerings for declarative models are much more limited. Even more so if the BPE needs to be able to handle decision logic captured in the models, which represents the knowledge that is so vital to the correct execution of loosely framed KiPs in real-life.

This work is part of a design science project and, more specifically, a design science cycle to develop the architecture of a business process management system for loosely framed KiPs. In previous work, we have created a modeling language specifically for this type of processes, called DeciClare (see chapter 2), and developed an automated framework for creating DeciClare models by way of process mining (see chapters 3 and 4). The contribution of this part of the chapter is a generic and high-level framework to support the execution of declarative process models with a data perspective. This is achieved by automatically generating sets of activities that are allowed, conditionally allowed and disallowed as the next activity at each point during the execution of the process. The framework is generic because it does not assume a specific modeling language, but rather a large family of languages that can satisfy the language requirements stated in this work. Consequently, the actual constraint validation techniques and corresponding computational complexity are out of scope as they are language depend. The goal is to pave the way for flexible decision- and process-aware support for loosely frame and KiPs.

The remainder of this first part of the chapter is structured as follows. Section 5.1.2 presents the research methodology used in this part of the chapter. The problem statement and the requirements for the solution artifact are presented in Sect. 5.1.3. In Sect. 5.1.4, the generic framework is proposed based on the requirements from Sect. 5.1.3. Subsequently, the DeciClare language is used to demonstrate a proof-of-concept implementation of the framework in the context of a realistic healthcare process in Sect. 5.1.5. Section 5.1.5.3 gives an overview of the related research on this topic. In Sect. 5.1.5.4 this part of the chapter is concluded and directions for future research are presented.

5.1.2 Research Methodology

This work applies the Design Science Research Methodology [38, 39] to develop a high-level framework to support the execution of declarative process models with a data perspective (i.e., the design artifact). The problem and requirements for the design artifact are defined in the next section. Because there is not a lot of literature on BPEs, the requirements are based on scattered information from literature, practical examples of BPEs from existing BPMSs and common-sense extensions of these principles.

The design artifact will be demonstrated by way of a prototype implementation. This should prove that a fully functional implementation of the framework is practically achievable and give an idea of how it would work.

5.1.3 Problem Statement and Solution Requirements

Declarative process models consist of many individual constraints and each of these constraints possibly applies to a different context. The result is that it can be very difficult for a user to quickly get an overview and find the process variation suitable for a certain process instance. This is largely due to the inherent nature of the processes being modeled, namely loosely framed KiPs. For example, consider the sheer number of possible diagnoses and treatments to the disposal of an emergency services doctor when a new patient arrives. The decision to follow a specific process variation is taken incrementally by the doctor during the process execution by choosing one or maybe a couple of activities to do next at a time. Because declarative models are hard to read or understand, there is no straightforward way in which they can be enacted directly by users.

A BPE is a software tool that offers supports the execution of a business process model. In this case, it should enact a declarative process model by creating a simplified summary for the users based on the specific process instance context. This summary will need to satisfy the following engine requirements (ER):

ER1. *The workflow control data containing the current state of each process instance (i.e., the already executed activities and used resources) should be available*

ER2. *The workflow relevant data of each process instance (e.g., age and gender of patient, presented symptoms...) should be available*

ER3. *All behavior allowed by the declarative model should be allowed*

ER4. *All behavior that violates the declarative model should be prohibited*

The four engine requirements above represent the foundation of a BPE; the typical responsibilities of a BPE in a BPMS in literature [3, 66, 83, 189] and the available real-life examples (e.g., jBPM[1], Activiti[2], DCR Graphs simulation engine[3], etc.). Depending on the expressive power of the declarative modeling language used to create the model, the resulting BPE can incorporate the control-flow, data and resource perspectives of the process. For loosely framed KiPs it remains essential that the freedom allowed by the given declarative model is not reduced by the BPE. The model does not need to be complete and the available constraints should be followed, but it should always present every option available according to the model. The BPE is not an expert system that replaces knowledge workers, but rather a tool to make their job easier.

To make the BPE more user-friendly, it would be useful to provide the user with an explanation of why certain activities are prohibited or will impose future restrictions and with some form of task list or description containing the constraints that still need to be satisfied by executing future activities. The following engine requirements are based on common sense extensions of the typical responsibilities of a BPE as described in literature [65, 190–192] and features real-life BPEs to improve the user-friendliness (e.g., the reminder functionality of Activity):

ER5. *The reasons why certain activities are not possible at certain times or in certain contexts should be available in the form of the constraint of the declarative model that would be violated*

ER6. *The restrictions that need to be dealt with later in the execution of the instance should be available to the users (e.g., execute activity X within 5 h)*

ER7. *A warning should be given for all behavior that potentially could lead to a live- or deadlock (prevention is even better, but not always computationally feasible depending on the used declarative process modeling language)*

BPEs require certain information about the process and its instances to be able to deliver useful results. Early BPEs were only concerned with the activities in a process and the relations between them [193]. Newer BPEs also add information about the resources involved in the process (e.g., personnel). ER1 and ER2 already require the BPE to keep track of the state and specific context of each process instance, but additional requirements are needed on the process model level to be able to create a data-aware declarative BPE. We summarized the informational needs in 8 language

---

[1] https://www.jbpm.org/

[2] www.activiti.org - Open Source Business Automation

[3] https://dcrsolutions.net/

requirements (LR). If the process modeling language used to create the process model does not support these LRs, it might be possible to provide this information separate from the model.

LR1. *A set of all activities of the process*

LR2. *A set of all resources involved in the process*

LR3. *A set of all data elements involved in the process*

LR4. *The capabilities of each resource (e.g., a dialysis machine can be simultaneously used in maximally two process instances)*

LR5. *The availability of each resource (i.e., how many of this type of resource and when they are available for a process instance)*

LR6. *The relationships that apply between resources (e.g., a nurse can take on the role of both a scrub nurse and an OR nurse)*

LR7. *The relationships that apply between the activities and/or the resources (e.g., the patient must be registered before doing an examination and doing an examination requires a doctor and an examination room)*

LR8. *The decision logic, based on the data elements from LR3, that governs the relationships from LR5 and LR6*

5.1.4   Data-Aware Declarative Process Enactment Framework

The ER1 and ER2 are related to the process instance and are stored on the enactment level. ER1 can be satisfied by keeping a history for each process instance of steps performed and resources utilized. ER1 requires access to the information system of the organization to get the necessary data values and real-time resource usage stats. This is not trivial in real-life, but for the purpose of this work we will assume that this data is directly available in the same format as defined in the declarative model.

The satisfactory execution of a process instance requires the joined efforts of the BPE and the knowledge workers of the process because declarative models do not define explicit pathways to follow. The BPE takes on the role of relevant information provider and the knowledge workers use this information to make the decision on what to do next. The framework at the core of the BPE consists of two phases. In the first phase, the BPE uses the workflow relevant and control data (ER1 and ER2) to calculate the parts of the declarative model that apply specifically to the executing instance by looking at the decision logic and preconditions for each constraint (see Table 5.23). Note that vacuously satisfied constraints [194] should be included (perhaps separately) as they convey important information on possible future restrictions. In the second phase, the BPE calculates which activities are available based on this relevant subset of the process model (see Table 5.24). It is then up to the knowledge workers to make the actual decision on how to proceed. The decision to execute a certain activity next will prompt an update of the workflow control data and likely generate additional data, which in turn triggers the BPE to redo the two phases. This is repeated until an ending is reached.

The second phase creates five (unsorted) sets of activities, which we will call tiers:

Table 5.1   The first phase of the framework of a declarative business process engine

#	Description	Req.
	Input: a declarative process model, the current state and current context of a process instance	
1.	Make a set of all constraints in the declarative model	LR1-LR8
2.	Check which constraints are active for the process instance by comparing the process instance data with the decision logic of the constraints. Remove the inactive constraints from the list.	ER1
3.	Remove all constraints for which the prerequisites are not satisfied by the history of executed activities and used resources of this process instance.	ER1
	Output: a set of all constraints applicable to the given process instance	

Table 5.2   The second phase of the framework of a declarative business process engine

	Input: a declarative process model and the output of the first phase
1.	Make set of all activities defined in the model, called the potential next-executed activities.
2.	For each activity in the set of potential next-executed activities:
	For each constraint from the set of applicable constraints:
	Validate that executing this potential next-executed activity would not violate the constraint.
	If only satisfied if executed after waiting a finite amount of time, store the constraint in the set of time-violated constraints for this potential next-executed activity.
	Else if only satisfied if future requirements are fulfilled, store the constraint in the set of activity-restricting constraints for this potential next-executed activity
	Else if only satisfied if the active resource (=current user of the system) is a different resource than the current active resource, store the constraint in the set of resource-restricting constraints for this potential next-executed activity.
	Else store constraint in the set of violated constraints for this potential next-executed activity.
3.	For each activity in the set of potential next-executed activities:
	If the violated constraints set is not empty, add activity to tier E.
	Else if the time-violated constraints set is not empty, add activity to tier D.
	Else if the resource-restricting constraints set is not empty, add activity to tier C.
	Else if the activity-restricting constraints set is not empty, add activity to tier B.
	Else add activity to tier A.
	Output: tiers A, B, C, D and E

(A) A set consisting of the activities that are available for execution as the next activity without any future restrictions applying.
(B) A set consisting of the activities that are available for execution as the next activity, but with future restrictions applying. These future restrictions come in the form of activities that are required or prohibited to be executed in the future so that the partial instance can be finished correctly.
(C) A set consisting of the activities that are available for execution as the next activity (i.e., tier A or B), but only if the active user is changed to another user.
(D) A set of the activities that are not available now but will be after a specified amount of time has elapsed (and will subsequently move to tier A or B).
(E) A set of the activities that are not available for execution as the next activity.

These five tiers give an overview of the allowed and prohibited behavior. ER3 and ER4 are satisfied by allowing only the activities in tiers A and B to be executed next. All activities in tier B are subject to restrictions that need to be dealt with later in the process. In contrast to the activities in tier A, the BPE cannot guarantee that the activities in tier B will not lead to a live- or deadlock. By placing them in a separate tier, this serves as a warning for the user to keep an eye on these restrictions (ER7).

ER5 calls for information to help the knowledge workers executing the process to understand why an activity is in a specific tier. To fulfill this requirement, each activity in tiers C, D and E will be accompanied with the constraints that would be violated by executing the activity next, which is a byproduct of the second step of the second phase. ER6 relates to the possible restrictions that apply to a certain partial instance and will need to be satisfied before the instance can finish in a correct way (e.g., X needs to be executed because Y has been executed). Fulfilling this requirement is a twofold process. Firstly, the constraints that result in these restrictions must be gathered. This set is already being composed as part of the second step of the second phase: the set of activity-restricting constraints. Secondly, the information needs to be made available to the user. The user needs to be able to view this set of restrictions, both for the current partial trace as well as for each activity from tier B (= the restrictions that would apply if this activity is selected as the next executed activity).

Additionally, some extra information about resource restrictions, time delays and deadlines that apply during the process execution can be added. Each activity in tiers C and D can be annotated with, respectively, the required user and the time delay that needs to be respected before it can move to tier A or B. The delay for a certain activity can be calculated by comparing the remainder of the current time minus the activation time, and the delays as specified by the constraints in the set of time-violated constraints for that activity from the second phase. Activities in tiers A and B can be annotated with the deadlines, if applicable, before which each activity needs to be executed. The relevant deadline can be calculated as the lowest deadline from the constraints in the set of activity-restricting constraints from the second step of the second phase, compared to the current time and taking into account the activation time of each of these constraints. Also, the subset of constraints from the full declarative model that apply to the current partial trace and for each activity in tier A and B can be made available, so that the user can review only those constraints that actually matter in this process instance. Again, we would preferably include the vacuously satisfied constraints separately, as these could be interesting when considering future restrictions.

Finally, there is one more possible scenario to be considered. As constraints can have deadlines before which they need to be satisfied, it is possible that a deadline is not satisfied (i.e., the necessary activities are not executed in time). This causes a deadlock. A BPE cannot directly prevent this, as user input is required for executing activities and it is the user's responsibility to monitor the deadlines as shown by the BPE.

5.1.5 Demonstration

As a proof-of-concept, we will use the DeciClare language to satisfy the language requirements from Sect. 5.1.3 and demonstrate a working implementation of the data-aware declarative process enactment framework proposed in the previous section.

5.1.5.1 Process Definition: DeciClare

DeciClare is a mixed-perspective declarative process and decision modeling language that specifically targets loosely framed KiPs (see chapter 2). It can be used to create detailed models of the control-flow, data and resource aspects of these processes. This work uses a direct instantiation (i.e., a temporary visual syntax in a textual format) of the abstract syntax, as a real visual syntax has not yet been developed at this time. The foundation of DeciClare is the Declare language and most of its extensions [22, 71, 84], which are either incorporated in a direct or generalized way. Therefore, Declare models can be easily converted to equivalent DeciClare models. Additionally, more perspectives were added as well as concepts from the DMN language [195]. The latter makes the resulting language 'data-aware', because data values can be used to (de)activate constraints based on the specific execution context, and capable of modeling the decision logic that typically governs KiPs. DeciClare supports 36 constraint templates (i.e., types of constraints) spanning four template classes: existence, relation, resource and data. 26 of these templates have time parameters expressing the time interval in which the constraint applies.

The implementation of the DeciClareEngine-tool presented in this work supports the 18 most important constraint templates of DeciClare (see Appendix F). A Deci-Clare model can contain all the information necessary to satisfy LR1-LR8 from Sect. 5.1.3. Activities, resources and all their relations can be fully modeled, and the constraints can be enriched with activation and deactivation decisions, based on the data elements, to allow for a level of detail that closely matches reality.

5.1.5.2   DeciClareEngine

The DeciClareEngine tool (github.com/stevmert/DeciClareBPMS/blob/master /engine/releases/DeciClareEngine.jar, the code can also be found on this GitHub) has been developed to demonstrate how the generic framework from Sect. 5.1.4 can be implemented. It is a data-aware declarative BPE that takes a DeciClare model as input. This means that it supports the control-flow, decision logic, time restrictions, resource authorizations and resource usages of the given process model.

When starting the BPE, the user first needs to select the role he or she will take on during the process instance before the main interface opens. At the top of the screen (left side of Fig. 5.30), the current time and user (= current resource) can be found as well as the current partial trace. The tiers A to E are displayed in the middle of the screen. And at the bottom of the screen, all data elements used in the model are listed with the option to add or change them for the current instance. The user can execute an activity from tier A or B by clicking on it. This prompts a screen where the user can enter the duration of the activity and change the data elements as part of the activity execution (right side of Fig. 5.30). The 'Explanation'-button next to the activities in tiers B, C, D and E presents the user with a set of the specific constraints that caused the activity to be placed in that specific tier (i.e., future restrictions or violations). Note that delays and deadlines are signaled next to the activity name and that their current status can be checked at any time as part of the explanation. To get the subset of constraints that are currently active, the user can click on the 'Relevant model'-button at the bottom of the screen or next to the corresponding

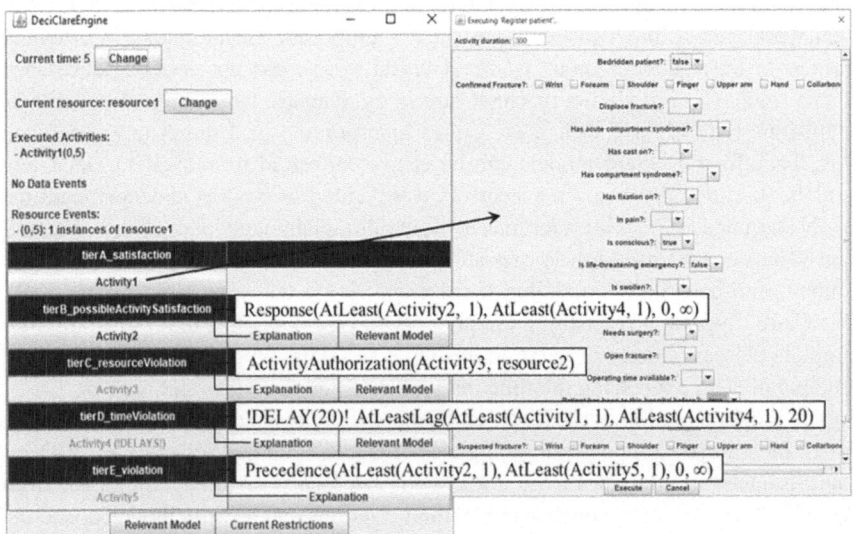

Fig. 5.1 The main interface (left), with added explanations, and the activity execution dialog (right)

activity. Vacuously satisfied constraints are included in this summary, although they are not yet displayed separately.

As the example model, we will use the healthcare process for treating arm-related fractures introduced in Sect. 2.5.1 (also see Appendix D). It is a realistic, but simplified, representation of the registration, diagnosis and treatment of patients with one or more (possible) fractures of the fingers, hands, wrists, forearms, upper arms, shoulders and collarbones in an emergency department of a hospital. The DeciClare model contains 229 constraints, of which 183 are supported by the current version of the tool. The process instance used to demonstrate the tool is of a 24-year-old woman who enters the emergency services with pain in her wrist after a bicycle accident. Every activity of the process is listed in the first column of Table 5.25. The other columns are snapshots (Sx) (i.e., 0–13) showing in which tier each activity was placed by the BPE at that time in the process.

S0 is the moment that the patient walks in the emergency room, with the receptionist as active user. The receptionist is not authorized to execute 7 of the 8 available activities, all of which come with future restrictions. The triage nurse takes a quick peek at the patient and concludes that her condition is not life-threatening, triggering the corresponding data event. This reduces the number of available activities to just one (S1), because only in the worst cases it is possible to skip the registration at the start. Next, the patient is registered at the reception, during which the receptionist sets the four data attributes relevant to the process (i.e., been to this hospital before, older than 14 years old, not bedridden and conscious) and the used resources (i.e., receptionist and reception desk). The user is currently asked to input the duration, data events and resource events of the executed activity (right side of Fig. 5.30), but in real settings this data should be extracted directly from the applications used to capture this data. Once registered, 7 activities become available, but the receptionist is only authorized to unregister the patient (S2). At this point, the active user is switched to a doctor, who is authorized to execute the 6 other activities (S3). By looking at the future restrictions that apply to the current partial instance, the doctor can see that several activities are now mandatory for this instance: unregistering the patient, taking a medical history, doing a clinical examination, taking an X-ray, applying ice, choosing a treatment and giving some pain relief. The doctor decides to proceed by letting a nurse take the patient's medical history, triggering two more data events (i.e., no current cast or fixation on the wrist in question) and one resource event (i.e., nurse used). Taking the medical history of the patient unlocks an additional activity in tier B: doing a clinical examination (S4). This is also the activity the doctor chooses to do next, which in turn triggers four more data events (i.e., suspected fracture of wrist, swollen, in pain and not an open fracture) and two resource events (i.e., uses doctor and exam room). S5 has 18 available activities. Because the doctor indicated that the patient is in pain, she can now receive some pain relief. After giving her a NSAID painkiller, 17 activities become available (S6). Note that prescribing anticoagulants is in tier D because there must be at least 12 h between receiving NSAID painkillers and receiving anticoagulants. 12 h later, this activity would move back to tier B.

By taking another look at the future restriction that currently apply, the doctor can see that three activities are still mandatory for this instance: unregistering the

Table 5.3 An overview of the activities and the tier in which they were placed for each snapshot

	Receptionist			Doctor									Receptionist	
	0	1	2	3	4	5	6	7	8	9	10	11	12	13
Register patient	B	**B**	E	E	E	E	E	E	E	E	E	E	E	E
Take medical history of patient	C	E	C	**B**	B	B	B	B	B	B	B	B	C	E
Clinical examination of patient	C	E	E	E	**B**	B	B	B	B	B	B	B	C	E
Doctor consultation	E	E	E	E	E	B	B	B	**B**	B	B	B	C	E
Take X-ray	E	E	E	E	E	B	B	**B**	B	B	B	B	C	E
Take CT scan	E	E	E	E	E	B	B	B	B	B	B	B	C	E
Prescribe NSAID painkillers	E	E	E	E	E	**B**	B	B	B	B	B	B	C	E
Prescribe SAID painkillers	E	E	E	E	E	B	B	B	B	B	B	B	C	E
Prescribe anticoagulants	E	E	E	E	E	B	D	D	D	D	D	D	D	E
Prescribe stomach protecting drug	E	E	E	E	E	B	B	B	B	B	B	B	C	E
Prescribe rest (= no treatment)	E	E	E	E	E	B	B	B	B	B	B	B	C	E
Apply ice	C	E	C	B	B	B	**B**	B	B	B	B	B	C	E
Apply cast	E	E	E	E	E	E	E	E	B	B	B	B	C	E
Remove cast	E	E	E	E	E	E	E	E	E	E	E	E	E	E
Apply splint	C	E	C	B	B	B	B	B	B	B	**B**	B	C	E
Apply sling	C	E	C	B	B	B	B	B	B	**B**	B	B	C	E
Apply fixation	E	E	E	E	E	E	E	E	B	B	B	B	C	E
Remove fixation	E	E	E	E	E	E	E	E	E	E	E	E	E	E
Apply bandage	C	E	C	B	B	B	B	B	B	B	B	B	C	E
Apply figure of eight bandage	E	E	E	E	E	E	E	E	B	B	B	B	C	E
Perform surgery	E	E	E	E	E	E	E	E	B	B	B	B	C	E
Apply intra-compartmental pressure monitor	E	E	E	E	E	B	B	B	B	B	B	B	C	E
Let patient rest	C	E	C	B	B	B	B	B	B	B	B	B	B	E
Stay in patient room	E	E	E	E	E	B	B	B	B	B	B	B	C	E
Unregister patient	E	E	B	C	C	C	C	C	C	C	C	C	**A**	E

patient, applying ice and taking an X-ray. The former is straightforward, but the latter two are due to the specific context of the case. Ice treatment is needed because the wrist is swollen and the X-ray to take a closer look at the patient's wrist. The doctor decides to do the ice treatment first. S7 offers the same options as the previous one and now the X-ray is selected, triggering two more resource events (i.e., nurse and X-ray room used). This results in four additional activities becoming available (S8). A doctor consultation to discuss the scan is now a mandatory, as stated in the current restrictions, so the doctor does this consultation next. During the consultation (using a doctor and an exam room), the doctor confirms the suspected wrist fracture by looking at the X-ray photo but, luckily, also that it is not a displaced or unstable fracture. This means that surgery is not required. The same activities are available in S9, yet it is now mandatory to apply a sling and a cast/splint in the future. The doctor decides to apply a splint next, which triggers another resource event (nurse used). Again, the same activities are available afterwards (S10). So now the doctor applies a sling to support the splinted wrist of the patient. In S11, the same activities are available, but the only current restriction now is that the patient will need to be unregistered in the future. The doctor decides that the patient can go home, so she is asked to go and unregister at the reception. The active user is now switched to the receptionist again (S12), which moves unregistering the patient from tier D to tier A (and 19 others from B to D). This means that no restrictions will remain after its execution. Finally, the receptionist unregisters the patient, triggering two more resource events (receptionist and reception desk used). No activities are available in S12, and the instance is in a conforming state according to the process model, so the user gets a message that the process has ended successfully.

5.1.5.3 Related Work

The existing BPEs can be classified according to the predictability-spectrum of the processes for which they are best suited. In this section, the differences between the DeciClareEngine-tool, used in the demonstration of this work, and each of the existing BPEs that target loosely framed processes will be highlighted in more detail.

The DECLARE framework is based on the Declare language [22], for which efficient techniques for the actual validation of (MP-)Declare constraints have been proposed [168]. Everything that can be expressed in Declare, can be expressed in the DeciClare language presented in chapter 2. Yet, the opposite is not true as DeciClare adds a data and resource perspective as well as an explicit concept of time in the form of deadlines and delays. So, compared to the DECLARE framework, DeciClareEngine additionally takes decision logic, resources, deadlines and delays into account. More recently, a BPE for the MP-Declare language was proposed that maps the constraints to Alloy and uses the corresponding satisfiability solver [196]. This approach can prevent live- and deadlocks. However, it is only feasible for very small models (e.g., 10 constraints) due to the computation complexity that results from the state space explosion. DeciClareEngine has no support for this yet, but this feature will be revisited in the future. Models of loosely framed KiPs are typically big and complex. Therefore, we will focus on investigating partial or heuristic versions of these features in future work.

ReFlex [197] is a BPE that uses a graph-based rule engine to overcome certain limitations of Linear Temporal Logic (LTL), as is used by the Declare language. It uses 7 types of edges that correspond to 6 constraint templates of Declare and 1 extra type of constraint. DeciClare, and therefore DeciClareEngine, also supports these 7 types of constraints and additionally offers support for time delays and deadlines, and a data and resource perspective. The selling point of ReFlex is also the detection of live- and deadlocks.

DCR Graphs have an online platform[4] that includes a BPE as part of the graph editor (for simulation). The DCR language has 6 relations (roughly equivalent to the Response and Precedence templates of DeciClare) and a clear visual syntax with support for hierarchical modeling. The simplicity of DCR Graphs is good for human understanding but limits its expressive power, although a data perspective [23] and some time-concepts (in DCR 2.0) have been added recently. DeciClare has additional support for more complex constraints, general context data elements, changing values of data attributes during the process execution and deadlines. On a functional level, the DCR Graphs BPE is quite similar to the prototype presented as demonstration of this work, albeit based on a less expressive language but with a much more polished interface. There is no academic description of how the DCR Graphs BPE works internally, although a demonstration is provided in Marquard et al. [198]. The contribution of this work is the generic framework to base this kind of BPE on, which has not been published before.

5.1.5.4   Conclusion and Future Research

This part of the chapter proposes a generic framework for creating data-aware declarative BPEs and demonstrates it by applying it to create a BPE for the DeciClare process modeling language. A BPE based on the proposed framework can support the execution of a real-life loosely framed KiPs, taking into account the control-flow, data and resource perspectives and corresponding decision logic governing them.

Due to the complexity and understandability issues of declarative languages, declarative models are seldom useful during the execution of processes. A BPE can be used to support the process actors during the execution of the process model by offering a process-aware view on what has been done already, what can or cannot be done next and what will need to or cannot happen in the future. The main advantage of using a BPE for the execution of a process is, of course, the certainty of conformance to a predefined process model. However, it can also be the foundation for a truly flexible information system, because it enables the rapid deployment of process changes in dynamic environments. Just make the necessary changes to the underlying process model. The BPE allows for these changes to be communicated to all

---

[4]https://dcrsolutions.net/

process actors and at the same time enforce that the changes are being implemented correctly.

In addition to offering runtime support, BPEs are also an essential tool for process simulation. Simulation makes it possible to analyze the impact of different runtime decisions or changes to the process model itself on the process outcome or characteristic. Another way to use model simulation, would be to validate a model that is the result of process mining or interviews. Historical or fictitious process instances can be simulated using the BPE, allowing domain experts to validate the process model in specific and more relatable contexts. This type of model validation is similar to how Benevides et al. [199] uses Alloy to simulate OntoUML models to validate that the model allows all wanted interpretations, while excluding the unwanted ones. It is also a powerful tool for educational purposes. The current education for doctors and other medical personnel leans heavily on internships so that the trainee can learn on the job from more experienced personnel. An educational simulator offers the trainee an additional tool to learn how things are done in a certain hospital and gain valuable experience in a risk-free environment. By using a mined process model that includes decision logic, it even has the potential to reveal (some of) the tacit knowledge of experienced colleagues to the trainee without a need for any direct interaction with those colleagues or patients.

The current design cycle of our research project is not finished yet. DeciClareEngine will be further refined by: 1) Adding support for the missing constraint templates and deactivation decisions, 2) Adding support for dynamic resource availabilities on process instance level, 3) Adding support for parallel execution of activities and 4) Investigating partial live- or deadlock detection or prevention mechanisms. A thorough comparison of the advantages and disadvantages of process execution with and without the use of DeciClareEngine is also planned for future research.

5.2   Comparing Strategies to Generate Experience-Based Clinical Process Recommendations that Leverage Similarity to Historic Data

5.2.1   Introduction

Healthcare processes can be subdivided into two groups: medical diagnosis/treatment processes and organizational/administrative processes [14]. We focus solely on the former. These kinds of processes are characterized as dynamic, multi-disciplinary, flexible, human-centric and knowledge-intensive processes [34, 137]. Consequently, the process actors executing the process (i.e., doctors and other medical personnel) are constantly confronted with decisions on what to do next from a large and diverse set of options. Decision making can be very demanding and even overwhelming, certainly for less experienced process actors. The current IT infrastructure remains lacking in support for decision making [200]. This is one of the reasons for requiring internships for new personnel. It gives them time to get a feel of how things are done in a certain department by following around more experienced personnel. However, these intern periods are time and effort consuming, not to mention expensive. Adding an additional channel for externalizing the knowledge of more experienced process actors as guidance, without them having to do anything extra, would have clear benefits [201]. Not only for less experienced process actors, but also for the other process actors. The result will be that the offered service will be more uniform, intern periods can be shortened, and process actors get relieved of some of the daily pressure.

In this second part of the chapter, we take the first step towards offering such guidance in the form of recommendations for flexible knowledge-intensive processes, and more specifically healthcare processes concerning the medical diagnosis and treatment of patients. The purpose of these recommendations is not to steer the process according to some optimization criteria, but rather to offer a direct reflection of the experience encapsulated in previous executions of the process. The results are returned to the users as process recommendations: a ranked list of the activities that are predicted to potentially be executed as the next activity and the corresponding probability estimations based on the most similar previously completed executions. The performance of a variety of strategies was measured and compared. The strategies can differ in what information they focus on, but they all leverage similarities between the currently executing process instance and the available historic data. The research questions (RQ) of this work are the following:

RQ1. Which prediction strategies perform well for knowledge-intensive and flexible healthcare processes?

RQ2. What kind of precision and consistency can be achieved and in what amount of computation time?

RQ3. How much data is needed to for near-optimal precision?

RQ4. Which strategies could be useful benchmarks to evaluate more advanced techniques (e.g., neural networks) in the future?

The strategies were implemented and applied to three different healthcare data sets: two real-life event logs and one artificial log. They are evaluated on the accuracy and consistency of the recommendation rankings (i.e., average accuracy, multi-class brier score, log loss and rank score) and the required computation time.

The remainder of this part of the chapter is structured as follows. Section 5.2.2 gives an overview of the related research. The relevant terminology and formal problem definition are presented in Sect. 5.2.3. In Sect. 5.2.4, the applied research methodology is presented. The prediction strategies used to generate recommendations are explained in Sect. 5.2.5. Section 5.2.6 describes the setup and results of experiments to evaluate the prediction strategies. The results of the experiments are discussed in Sect. 5.2.7. And finally, this part of the chapter is concluded and directions for future research are suggested in Sect. 5.2.8.

5.2.2   Related Work

The domain of process recommendations as a way to offer guidance to the process actors is still in its infancy. The prediction, ranking and probability estimation of potential next activities as a direct reflection of the experience encapsulated in previous executions of the process is, to the best of our knowledge, yet to be tackled. However, process recommendations have been proposed with other goals in mind. Schonenberg and Weber [202] use three different trace abstractions to generate recommendations based on historic executions that minimize the cycle time of a partially executed process instance. The trace abstractions (prefix, set and multi-set) have also been used in this work. Barba et al. [203] propose a recommendation system for process-aware information systems that generate an enactment plan for the remainder of a partially executed process instance using constraint-based approach with a declarative process model as input. The differences with this work are that only one enactment plan is proposed at any one time, so no more than one recommended next activity per available resource (i.e., no ranking), and an enactment plan specifies the remainder of the process instance (i.e., all recommended remaining activities in a specified order). The enactment plans are also optimized according the performance goals of the process, whereas the goal of this work is to reflect the current way of working.

The related domain of predictive process monitoring is concerned with the continuous generation of predictions (often referred to as next-element predictions) of what activities should be performed and what input data values to provide, so that the likelihood of violation of business constraints is minimized [204, 205]. A business constraint can be a business goal, a desired outcome or a range for a key performance indicator (KPI) (e.g., instance duration should be less than 24 h). The prediction of the next, the last or all remaining activities as well as the similarity to previously executed instances is used to estimate the likelihood of compliance based on the current state of the instance and the available historic data. The key difference to this work is that the goal of predictive process monitoring is typically to indicate when special attention, or even an intervention, is needed to prevent the process instances from reaching an undesirable state. So, the prediction of the likelihood of compliance to some predicated constraint is of primary concern, more so than the precision of the next-activity prediction. Therefore, the prediction of the next activity is typically just a means to an end and not necessarily conveyed to the process actors. In this work, our focus is solely on the prediction, ranking and probability estimation of potential next activities as a direct reflection of the experience encapsulated in previous executions of the process and we make no attempt to optimize the likelihood of achieving some business goal or to keep some KPI within an optimal range. In real-life applications, the ranking and probability estimations of the potential next activities proposed in this work would be made available to process actors as a form of guidance. As a result, the primary focus is on the precision of the predictions as well as the relative ranking and the robustness of the ranking. Some predictive process monitoring systems can also provide recommendations as a way of intervening when potential goal violations loom. This is an attempt to sway the process actor to follow historic executions that do satisfy the predicated constraint, as opposed to other historic executions that do not. The difference here is that they value certain similar historic executions more than others based on their outcomes, as opposed to just the direct similarity between the current execution and historic executions as is the goal of this work.

Several techniques used in predictive process monitoring could be useful in the context of this work, but it is difficult to compare the results from those papers with ours as the evaluation setup and criteria are different and the implementation, if available, often needs some adjustments to align it with the goals of this work. Di Francescomarino et al. [206] apply a clustering technique and a classifier to estimate whether a given predicate will be satisfied upon completion of an executing process instance. Evermann et al. [207] use recurrent neural networks with long short-term memory to predict the remaining time to completion and the next activity of partially executed process instances and Tax et al. [208] further investigated its applicability. van der Spoel et al. [185] use process mining techniques to predict the next activity and a classifier to predict future cost and duration of a partially executed process instance.

Another related domain is that of trace clustering. Trace clustering techniques are often applied to create clusters of similar completed process executions before process mining techniques are applied to create a model of each cluster. These techniques should not be applied to cluster a partially executed instance in clusters of completed executions, as this is a completely different problem. However, some techniques use traces abstractions as a first step towards comparing the similarity of traces and we have implemented several of these as strategies in this work. From Song et al. [209] we used the activity and transition trace profiles, which make abstraction of a trace by keeping only a set (or vector/matrix) of activities executed or activity transitions used in the trace. From De Leoni et al. [210] we used the control-flow manipulations CFP1 (i.e., the number of executions of a certain activity up to that point in the trace) and CFP3 (i.e., the activity transitions up to that point in the trace) as abstractions of a trace. Additionally, many cluster distance measures can be also be used as similarity metrics. We started from the distance measures in Song et al. [211] (e.g., Euclidean, Jaccard...) and added several others from different sources. The resulting strategies in a way make just one cluster with the abstraction of the partially executed instance as center. To calculate cluster distance (i.e., the similarity) between a partial and a completed instance, we introduced the concept of a variable-position similarity scorer.

5.2.3 Terminology and Formal Problem Definition

First, some explanations of terms or abbreviations that will be used throughout the remainder of this chapter (also see Table 12 and Table 18 for more terminology explanations):

- *Prediction points in a trace*: a trace is divided into prediction points, each coming right after the completion of an activity and one just before the start of the first activity in the trace. For example, a trace <A, B> has three prediction points: before A, after A and after B. For simplicity, we did not consider each moment in time between the execution of activities as a separate prediction point.
- *Position in a trace*: each prediction point in a trace has a position. Consequently, the prediction point before the execution of the first activity is position 0, after the execution of the first activity is position 1, and so on.
- *Multiset*: a set in which elements are not necessarily unique (i.e., a list without a specified order).
- *NextActs*: the set of potential next activities for every prediction point. Let *NextActs* $= [A_1,..., A_a, A_{a+1}]$ with a the number of executable activities and A_{a+1} representing the end of the trace (i.e., no more activities executed).
- *HT* (= historic trace): a trace of a previously completed process instance. The set of historic traces is used by the scorers to calculate recommendations for new partial traces. This set is also referred to as the learning set. Let $H = [HT_1,..., HT_k]$ with k the number of traces in the learning set and $HT_i = [A_{HTi(1)},..., A_{HTi(m)}, A_{a+1}]$ with m the number of executed activities in trace HT_i.
- *HPT* (= historic partial trace): a partial version of a HT where the activity and data events after a certain position in the *HT* are not considered.
- *CPT* (= current partial trace): the partial trace for which the recommendations are being calculated. Let $CPT = [A_{CPT(1)},..., A_{CPT(n)}]$ with n the number of already performed activities.

Now then we can provide a formal problem definition:

For each prediction point, predict $A_{CPT(n+1)} = [P_1, P_2,..., P_{a+1}]$ as a set of probability estimates for each potential next activity in *NextActs* given H so that $A_{CPT(n+1)}$ matches the as-is process as close as possible. $A_{CPT(n+1)}$ can subsequently be used to rank the activities of *NextActs*.

5.2.4 Research Methodology

The strategies described in the next section are the result of a literature review and some creativity. The literature review started from terms like 'process recommendation', 'recommender' and 'prediction strategies'. This led to papers on process recommendations and the domain of predictive process monitoring, but also more general and non-process-aware domains. The snowball method was followed to explore the latter, leading to relevant trace clustering techniques, general clustering techniques and string similarity measures. However, most of these were not directly applicable to the process recommendation context. Therefore, we created the heuristic proposed in Sect. 5.2.5.3 to allow these techniques to be applied to this context. Finally, we applied some creativity to find all possible uses for each strategy/measure and added of our own ideas, inspired by related literature. Of course, it should be noted that we excluded a class of potential strategies: black-box strategies (e.g., NN). This is planned as a follow-up comparison between the strategies discussed in this work and black-box strategies.

We will perform two major experiments using three different healthcare event logs to answer the research question from Sect. 5.2.1. The first experiment will compare the general predictive power of each of the strategies in order to answer RQ1, RQ2 and RQ4. The second experiment fill focus on the evolution of the predictive power of the strategies relative to the number of traces available to learn from. This should provide an answer to RQ3.

5.2.5 Strategies

We have identified 40 strategies to generate next-activity recommendations that all leverage trace similarity in one way or another. Most of these strategies have their roots in the related literature that came up when searching for topics like trace similarity, trace clustering, predictive process monitoring and vector/matrix similarity. We generalized, applied the same idea to other concepts and extrapolated some of those existing strategies to come up with additional strategies. And finally, we used our own creativity and domain knowledge to come up with the four more strategies (i.e., ActivityWithBefores, DataStateCustomOverlap and the combined strategies). We purposefully avoided more advanced techniques like neural networks, because of transparency concerns related to their black-box nature. However, in the future we will perform a comparison, including such advanced techniques, to evaluate if they can beat the strategies from this work and whether the loss of transparency would be worth any potential added precision.

Each strategy was implemented in what we will refer to as a similarity scorer. These scorers take H and a CPT as input and return a list of potential next activities ranked according to their corresponding probability estimates. A scorer can therefore be regarded as the brains of an eventual recommendation system, with the other components being responsible for the integration of the recommendation system in the electronic health record system and for the user interface to convey the results to the users. The scorers are split into three general classes: pre-calculated, positionless and variable-position similarity scorers. Some of the scorers use certain weights and other parameter settings to function properly. The hyperparameter values used in the experiments are given below. Note that these values were determined intuitively before running any experiments (i.e., guesstimates), but special attention was payed to keeping these values consistent across similar strategies. Small scale experiments ex post facto indicated that small variations in the hyperparameter values had little impact on the relative performance of the different strategies. However, there certainly is room for optimization through tuning.

5.2.5.1 Pre-calculated Similarity Scorers

These scorers calculate a frequency table once from H and use this table to generate a ranking of potential next activities and a corresponding probability estimate for the *CPT*. The computation times for these scorers presented in the experiments ignore the computation time of the frequency table, as this is a one-time cost (with a duration of just a couple of milliseconds).

- AbsoluteFrequency (=proportional guessing from Tax et al. [212]): calculates the absolute frequency in H of each activity in *NextActs*.
- ActivityInTraceFrequency (=set abstraction from Schonenberg and Weber [202]): calculates the frequency of each activity in *NextActs* as the percentage of traces from H in which it occurs at least once.
- RespondedFrequency (=similar to CFP3 from De Leoni et al. [210]): calculates for each activity in *NextActs*, and also for the start of trace, the frequency that it is directly followed by a certain other activity from *NextActs* in the traces of H. The size of the frequency table increases quadratically with the number of activities.
- StepFrequency (=Prefix abstraction from Schonenberg and Weber [202]): calculates the frequency of each activity in *NextActs* for each possible position as used in H.

5.2.5.2 Positionless Similarity Scorers

These scorers calculate the similarity at runtime between the *CPT* and the completed traces in H, so they do not consider any partial versions of the traces in H.

- IntraTraceFrequency (=multi-set abstraction from Schonenberg and Weber [202]): calculates a percentage for each activity in *NextActs* as the number of traces in H that have more occurrences of the activity than the *CPT*, divided the sum of this number for all activities in *NextActs*.
- IntraTraceFrequencyNotNull: the same as the IntraTraceFrequency scorer, but without considering the end of the trace as a separate activity. The thought process was that adding this extra activity, which occurs eventually in every *HT*, might be detrimental to the performance of the IntraTraceFrequency scorer because the added activity will potentially result in a higher rank and a lower probability estimate of the recommendation of the correct next activity for each prediction point except for the last one of a trace.

5.2.5.3 Variable-Position Similarity Scorers

These scorers calculate the similarity of the *CPT* with a *HT* by calculating the similarity of the *CPT* with all possible *HPTs* of a *HT* that stop in different positions. The similarity is not necessarily calculated for all possible *HPTs* of a *HT*, but rather heuristically. The current position in the *CPT* (i.e., the number of activities already executed for the *CPT*) is used as a starting point, and various positions left and right of the start position are considered until the stop criteria is reached for each direction. This criteria states that the search is stopped if there is no local improvement in the scores of 4 consecutive *HPTs* in that direction. After calculating the similarity score for each trace in *H*, the 100 most similar *HTs* are kept for calculating the probability estimates of the potential next activities. This '100' and '4' are parameters that can be further tuned in the future.

- UniqueActivity: calculates the similarity as the number of unique activities that were executed in both (partial) traces divided by the total number of unique activities executed in the *CPT*, minus a penalty of 0.001 times the number of unique activities that differ between both traces.
- Activity (= activity trace profile from Song et al. [209] and CFP1 from De Leoni et al. [210]): calculates the similarity as the weighted sum of two subscores, minus two penalty factors. The first subscore (weight = 0.7857) is the number of unique activities that were executed in both traces divided by the total number of unique activities executed in the *CPT*. The second subscore (weight = 0.2143) is the complement of the sum of the absolute differences between the number of repeated executions of shared activities of both traces, divided by the total number of activities executed in the *CPT*. The penalty factors are 0.001 times the number of unique activities not shared among both traces and 0.0001 times the number of repeated executions of activities that are not shared.
- ActivityWithBefores: calculates the similarity as the weighted sum of the Activity similarity score (weight = 0.7) and the complement of the sum of the differences in the before-relations of both traces, divided by the sum of the before-relations of the *CPT* (weight = 0.3). The before-relations of a trace consist of a set of activities, with corresponding number of occurrences, for each activity executed in the trace. The list contains all activities that were executed before the corresponding activity was executed. If an activity was executed multiple times, the list of its before-relation will be the sum of the activities executed before each execution.
- UniqueActivityTransition: calculates the similarity as the number of unique activity transitions that are part of both traces, divided by the total number of unique activity transitions in the *CPT*, minus a penalty of 0.001 times the number of unique activity transitions that differ between both traces. The transition from 'null' to the first activity is included.
- ActivityTransition (= transition trace profile from Song et al. [209]): calculates the similarity as the weighted sum of two subscores, minus two penalty factors. The first subscore (weight = 0.7857) is the number of unique activity transitions that are part of both traces, divided by the total number of unique activity transitions in the *CPT*. The second subscore (weight = 0.2143) is the complement of the sum of the absolute differences between the number of repetitions of activity transitions that are part of both traces, divided by the total number of activity transitions in the *CPT*. The penalty factors are 0.001 times the number of unique activity transitions not shared among both traces and 0.0001 times the number of repeated activity transitions that are not shared among both traces.

- DataStateCustomOverlap: calculates the similarity as the number of shared currently active data attributes in both traces, divided by the total number of currently active data attributes in the *CPT*, minus a penalty of 0.01 times the number of unique activities that differ between both traces.

We also considered the following general mathematical distance and similarity metrics (Euclidian and Jaccard from Song et al. [211], Tanimoto from Bajusz et al. [213] and the others were taken from the SimMetrics Java library, https://github.com/ Simmetrics, on the condition that they could be easily applied in this context):

- *Dice*: defined as twice the size of the intersection of two sets divided by sum of sizes of each separate set. Also known as the Sørensen index or Sørensen-Dice coefficient.
- *Jaccard*: defined as the size of the intersection of two sets divided by the size of the union of the sets.
- *Overlap Coefficient*: is defined as the size of the intersection of two sets divided by the size of the set that originates from the *CPT*.
- *Tanimoto Coefficient*: defined as the cosine of the angle between two sets expressed as sparse vectors.
- *Block Distance*: defined as the sum of the absolute differences of the Cartesian coordinates of two multisets. Also known as taxicab geometry, rectilinear distance, L1 distance, snake distance, city block distance, Manhattan distance or Manhattan length.
- *Euclidean Distance*: defined as the "ordinary" straight-line distance between two multisets in Euclidean space.
- *Simon White*: same as Dice, but with multisets.
- *Generalized Jaccard*: same as Jaccard, but with multisets.
- *Generalized Overlap Coefficient*: same as Overlap Coefficient, but with multisets.
- *Cosine Similarity*: Tanimoto Coefficient, but with multisets.

These metrics can calculate the distance or similarity between two (multi-)sets. A trace can be converted to such a (multi-)set abstraction by, for example, creating a (multi-)sets of all activities executed in that trace (similar the abstraction used by the UniqueActivity and Activity scorers). For each of these distance measures and similarity metrics we defined two scorers, and an additional third for all but the Simon White, Generalized Jaccard, Generalized Overlap Coefficient and Cosine Similarity metrics (as these would coincide with the non-multiset versions of the corresponding metric scorers):

- Activity...Scorer: the lists of activities events of the *CPT* and *HPT* are converted to (multi-) sets to calculate the metric.
- Data...Scorer: the lists of data events of the *CPT* and *HPT* are converted to (multi-) sets to calculate the metric.
- DataState...Scorer: the data states of the *CPT* and *HPT* are converted to (multi-) sets to calculate the metric. The data state is the set of data attributes that are active at the current point in the trace. So, it starts from the same (multi-)set as the Data...Scorer but removes all inactive data values.

5.2.5.4   Combinated Scorers

The scorers above all use an abstraction of just one aspect of the trace. Of course, the eventual goal is to create a scorer that takes multiple aspects into account. As an example of this, we also implemented two scorers that combine several of the aforementioned scorers.

- ActivityWithBeforesAndData: calculates the similarity as the weighted sum of two subscores. The first subscore is the ActivityWithBefores score (weight = 0.6) and the other is the DataStateCustomOverlap score (weight = 0.4).
- ActivityWithBeforesAndDataAndKBs: calculates a score for each potential next activity as a weighted combination of 5 scorers: ActivityWithBefores, DataState-CustomOverlap, RespondedFrequency, StepFrequency and AbsoluteFrequency. The first two are used to calculate a similarity score just like the ActivityWithBe-foresAndData scorer, but with slightly different weights (weight of ActivityWith-Befores = 0.4/0.59 and weight of DataStateCustomOverlap = 0.19/0.59). The final score is then calculated as the sum of ActivityWithBeforesAndData score (weight = 0.59), the RespondedFrequency score (weight = 0.4), the StepFre-quency score (weight = 0.009) and the AbsoluteFrequency score (weight = 0.001).

5.2.6   Experiments

We performed two experiments to compare the performance of the different strate-gies. The first experiment tries to answer RQ1, RQ2 and RQ4 by applying the scorers to three healthcare data sets and comparing the performance of the strategies on different types of data sets. The second experiment is similar, but it varies the size of H to investigate the relation between the predictive power and the size of H to answer RQ3.

5.2.6.1   Experiment 1: Comparing the General Predictive Power Over Different Data Sets

5.2.6.1.1 Experimental Setup
Three healthcare event logs were used:

- ArmFractures[5]: an artificial event log containing 5000 traces (31980 activity and 45147 data events using 9 unique activities and 21 unique data values to form traces of up to 11 activity events) about patients with suspected arm fractures. It spans parts of the hospital emergency and orthopedic departments and was created via interviews with domain experts.

---

[5]https://github.com/stevmert/EventLogs/blob/master/armFractures(5000)v2.zip

- Sepsis[6]: a real-life event log containing 1050 traces (15214 activity and 32885 data events using 16 unique activities and 214 unique data values to form traces of up to 185 activity events) specifically about sepsis cases that were extracted from the Enterprise Resource Planning system of a hospital.
- EmergencyDepartment: a real-life event log containing 41657 traces (625758 activity and 1350465 data events using 116 unique activities and 951 unique data values to form traces of up to 128 activity events) about the registration, triage, diagnosis and treatment of patients in the medical emergency department of the Belgian AZ Maria Middelares hospital. We are not at liberty to make this event log public due to a confidentiality agreement.

These event logs contain activity events as well as the relevant data events with the corresponding data values entered by the medical personnel during the execution of the process. The logs can all be categorized as flexible knowledge-intensive processes, but they do differ in how extreme they exhibit these properties. The EmergencyDepartment-log is the most complex data set, yet, it also has the most traces and details for the scores to base their recommendations on.

In this experiment, each scorer was used to calculate recommendations for each prediction point of each trace from the log with all other traces from that log as H. The experiments ran on an Intel Xeon Gold 6140 with 32 GB of RAM. The 36-cores were used to calculate the similarity scores of up to 36 traces from H in parallel. The results are evaluated using the trace-wise averages (i.e., for each trace, the average over all of its prediction points is calculated and the average of each of these traces scores is the final average) of four performance measures (see next paragraph), as opposed to the overall averages. Both averages will give similar results, but the overall averages have the undesired effect of giving longer traces a relatively higher weight because they have more prediction points. The longer traces are typically also harder to predict. Hence, they would skew the results. Trace-wise averages are more representational for general performance.

Three well-known classification performance measures were used to evaluate the performance of the scorers: *accuracy*, *log loss* and *multi-class brier score* [214]. These measures quantify the precision of the recommendations (RQ1 and RQ2) by comparing, respectively, the highest ranked recommendation, probability estimate of the highest ranked recommendation and probability estimates of each recommendation to the actual next activity. This gives us a lot of information on the relative predictive power of each strategy. However, the purpose of recommendations in this work is not merely to predict, but also as a tool to offer guidance to process actors. Therefore, we opted to define an additional performance measure that scores the consistency of the ranking of recommendations (RQ2): the *rank score*. Where the classification performance measures just make a distinction between right and wrong (e.g., ranked first), the rank score makes a distinction between levels of 'wrong'. For example, ranking the correct next activity as second or 15th makes a big practical

---

[6]Original Sepsis log: https://data.4tu.nl/repository/uuid:915d2bfb-7e84-49ad-a286-dc35f063a460
Sepsis log used in this paper (with preprocessed data): https://github.com/stevmert/EventLogs/blob/master/SepsisCases.zip

difference as process actors cannot be expected to consider much more than a few recommendations at the top.

The rank score is calculated as follows:

$$Rank\ score = \left(\sum\nolimits_{i=1}^{c} f_i r_i\right)^2$$

With c denoting the number of prediction outcomes/classes (i.e., the size of *NextActs*), f_i representing whether activity i was the correct next activity (i.e., $f_i \in \{0, 1\}$ and $f_i = 1$ iff activity i was the correct next activity) and r_i representing the ranking of potential next activity i.

The ideal rank score is equal to one, as this means that the correct next activity was ranked as first. Sub-optimal rankings will result in a rank score of more than one. The formula is squared so that worse rankings are exponentially penalized. This puts strategies that consistently have the correct next activity at the top of the ranking at an advantage.

5.2.6.1.2 Computational Results

The results of experiment 1 are summarized in Table 5.26 (these results and additional details are available at https://github.com/stevmert/recommendationExperiments). The average rank of the correct next activity is also included, as this is a more relatable than the quite abstract performance measures.

By design, the pre-calculated scorers are the fastest. But it is noteworthy that even the slowest scorer only needed an average of little more than 0.6 s of computation time for even the biggest and most complex event log (RQ2).

The color-coding of the table reveals that the results for the different performance measures are clearly correlated. A relatively good result for one measure usually also indicates relatively good performance for the others. In general, the variable-position activity similarity scorers come out on top. Their performance was consistently among the best for all logs. The differences between the different activity similarity scorers are small, but the Activity and ActivityWithBefores scorers consistently perform just slightly better (RQ1). The data and data state variable-position similarity scorers perform poorly across the board. This is not a big surprise, as predicting next activities without knowing what activities have already been performed is inherently more difficult. The gap is smaller for the data state scorers on the data-heavy EmergencyDepartment log. The performance of the positionless similarity scorers is below average. The distinction between the IntraTraceFrequency and IntraTraceFrequencyNotNull scorers was made due to concerns about the impact of adding the end of trace prediction. The results show that these concerns were legitimate. The IntraTraceFrequencyNotNull scorer has a higher accuracy for all logs compared to the IntraTraceFrequency scorer, however, the trade-off is a much higher log loss and rank score.

The performance of the pre-calculated scorers is a bit of a mixed bag. The AbsoluteFrequency and ActivityInTraceFrequency scorers perform poorly, the StepFrequency scorer performs average and the performance of the RespondedFrequency

Table 5.4 The results for experiment 1. For each column, the top performer is formatted in italics and bold and a color-coding was used to represent the best-to-worse ranking (green-yellow-red)

Scorer	AmiFractures						Sepsis						EmergencyDepartment					
	Calculation Time (ms)	Rank	Accuracy	Brier Score	Log Loss	Rank Score	Calculation Time (ms)	Rank	Accuracy	Brier Score	Log Loss	Rank Score	Calculation Time (ms)	Rank	Accuracy	Brier Score	Log Loss	Rank Score
AbsoluteFrequency	0.02	3.64	23.20%	0.0857	2.698	17.90	0.02	4.99	17.51%	0.0529	3.375	36.04	0.12	7.15	18.63%	0.0079	4.015	101.88
ActivityInTraceFrequency	0.01	3.62	14.11%	0.0860	2.935	19.50	0.01	5.63	8.36%	0.0534	3.554	40.30	0.11	7.22	8.29%	0.0079	4.110	99.97
StepFrequency	0.01	1.48	74.00%	0.0335	1.004	3.17	0.02	2.47	47.52%	0.0375	2.295	10.15	0.07	4.66	39.17%	0.0058	2.806	64.62
RespondedFrequency	0.01	1.34	80.98%	0.0268	0.750	2.55	0.01	2.28	57.15%	0.0331	1.959	9.80	0.07	3.43	55.43%	0.0047	2.147	44.44
IntraTraceFrequencyNotNull	4.72	2.45	57.25%	0.0786	8.342	12.08	0.01	3.11	43.43%	0.0509	6.531	26.48	15.04	6.42	37.09%	0.0078	7.520	1218.41
IntraTraceFrequency	2.33	2.33	54.11%	0.0337	2.273	6.67	1.84	3.35	38.36%	0.0509	3.088	13.29	106.75	6.42	37.09%	0.0077	3.960	114.86
ActivityBlockDistance	20.37	1.19	87.20%	0.0174	0.461	1.75	3.65	1.79	62.53%	0.0282	1.674	5.37	190.64	4.28	54.74%	0.0049	2.917	114.88
ActivityDice	15.06	1.41	78.86%	0.0174	0.461	1.75	3.53	1.79	58.09%	0.0306	1.828	6.07	248.49	4.45	54.74%	0.0049	2.917	122.90
ActivityEuclideanDistance	21.79	1.19	87.39%	0.0173	0.459	3.17	3.57	1.80	61.83%	0.0287	1.754	6.07	175.71	4.34	54.72%	0.0049	3.042	127.91
ActivityJaccard	15.63	1.45	78.86%	0.0319	2.332	3.17	3.35	1.89	58.00%	0.0306	1.824	7.48	163.56	4.45	54.62%	0.0048	2.829	111.10
ActivityOverlapCoefficient	17.43	1.41	78.43%	0.0322	2.382	3.41	3.37	2.14	50.58%	0.0345	1.980	7.48	205.86	3.92	52.76%	0.0049	2.506	81.94
ActivityTanimotoCoefficient	18.99	1.41	78.86%	0.0319	2.332	3.17	3.24	1.90	57.97%	0.0306	1.829	6.07	205.75	3.92	52.75%	0.0049	2.506	122.73
ActivityCosine	20.26	1.19	87.34%	0.0174	0.461	3.49	3.17	1.78	62.42%	0.0281	1.682	6.07	204.43	3.92	54.73%	0.0049	2.829	122.61
ActivityGeneralizedJaccard	20.28	1.19	78.86%	0.0173	0.461	1.75	3.17	1.78	62.54%	0.0281	1.674	5.33	242.56	4.37	54.43%	0.0049	2.953	128.61
ActivityGeneralizedOverlapCoefficient	20.61	1.25	82.72%	0.0215	0.577	2.02	3.93	2.04	55.48%	0.0327	1.915	5.33	191.18	3.92	54.75%	0.0048	2.576	95.49
ActivitySimonWhite	20.44	1.19	87.23%	0.0174	0.461	1.75	3.83	1.79	62.52%	0.0282	1.806	5.37	208.11	4.28	54.74%	0.0048	2.916	124.88
UniqueActivity	20.78	1.41	78.92%	0.0319	2.332	3.17	3.54	1.88	58.11%	0.0307	1.824	5.37	224.19	4.28	53.26%	0.0048	2.699	111.02
Activity	23.93	1.19	87.42%	0.0172	0.459	1.74	9.48	1.80	62.28%	0.0281	1.754	5.59	215.11	4.16	55.06%	0.0047	2.777	118.37
ActivityUniqueTransition	18.72	1.22	86.95%	0.0186	0.851	2.03	4.78	2.03	56.44%	0.0321	2.068	7.22	230.44	4.76	53.87%	0.0049	3.179	153.97
ActivityTransition	18.77	1.19	87.99%	0.0167	0.446	1.74	4.16	2.03	56.69%	0.0321	2.013	7.22	242.56	4.75	54.26%	0.0048	2.777	118.37
ActivityWithBefores	19.36	1.18	88.16%	0.0166	0.444	1.71	11.91	1.82	61.58%	0.0289	1.768	5.61	248.14	4.13	57.32%	0.0046	2.798	123.14
DataDice	40.52	1.18	88.16%	0.0166	0.788	1.71	4.94	4.46	30.07%	0.0547	12.135	34.74	188.10	21.28	27.63%	0.0086	15.701	1211.74
DataJaccard	20.73	3.47	45.07%	0.0870	18.788	19.00	5.00	4.66	30.04%	0.0547	12.141	34.75	181.28	21.27	27.63%	0.0085	15.686	1211.76
DataOverlapCoefficient	21.22	3.47	45.02%	0.0870	18.787	19.00	4.27	3.78	29.91%	0.0525	7.414	25.13	180.89	21.28	28.39%	0.0086	15.701	1211.76
DataTanimotoCoefficient	21.61	1.41	44.23%	0.0319	19.433	18.90	3.78	4.27	29.78%	0.0547	12.138	34.75	179.98	28.72	28.70%	0.0099	25.118	1692.17
DataBlockDistance	21.57	3.47	45.07%	0.0892	18.783	19.00	4.99	4.88	30.04%	0.0547	12.208	34.85	336.77	21.28	27.63%	0.0086	15.701	1211.76
DataCosineSimilarity	23.09	3.47	45.07%	0.0870	18.783	19.00	9.26	4.46	29.77%	0.0547	12.206	34.75	187.18	21.28	27.63%	0.0086	15.701	1211.76
DataEuclideanDistance	22.69	3.47	45.06%	0.0870	18.783	19.00	8.55	4.48	28.66%	0.0554	12.069	37.81	331.08	18.27	18.27%	0.0077	14.170	1692.21
DataGeneralizedJaccard	23.31	1.19	45.04%	0.0870	19.000	19.00	9.16	4.66	30.08%	0.0547	12.139	34.74	635.85	21.46	19.79%	0.0099	23.518	2518.??
DataGeneralizedOverlapCoefficient	22.39	3.47	45.02%	0.0870	18.787	19.00	4.66	4.66	30.08%	0.0547	12.196	34.74	188.59	21.27	28.39%	0.0085	15.587	1211.79
DataSimonWhite	22.51	3.49	45.07%	0.0892	19.433	18.90	5.58	3.78	29.92%	0.0547	7.413	25.12	198.08	11.78	37.70%	0.0062	8.099	590.49
DataStateJaccard	22.71	3.47	45.05%	0.0870	18.787	19.00	3.78	4.46	30.03%	0.0547	12.196	34.74	199.42	21.77	28.39%	0.0086	15.701	1211.79
DataStateDice	22.75	3.50	44.98%	0.0870	18.659	19.45	4.47	3.78	35.70%	0.0495	5.711	20.12	204.81	21.28	27.63%	0.0086	15.701	501.00
DataStateOverlapCoefficient	22.88	3.50	45.01%	0.0863	18.671	19.45	4.10	3.37	35.67%	0.0495	5.710	20.12	207.85	10.05	45.24%	0.0057	7.529	501.00
DataStateTanimotoCoefficient	23.17	3.52	43.93%	0.0879	18.659	19.45	3.43	3.37	35.70%	0.0495	5.711	20.12	206.55	9.40	45.67%	0.0057	6.763	460.14
DataStateBlockDistance	23.23	3.52	45.00%	0.0863	18.671	19.45	3.83	3.38	35.57%	0.0496	6.364	21.65	208.01	10.20	44.97%	0.0057	7.417	530.36
DataStateEuclideanDistance	24.85	3.50	45.01%	0.0863	18.671	19.45	6.52	3.37	35.66%	0.0495	5.711	20.12	426.20	10.05	45.21%	0.0057	7.417	501.00
DataStateCustomOverlap	25.09	3.50	44.98%	0.0863	18.671	19.45	6.70	3.41	35.39%	0.0496	5.827	20.58	631.70	10.05	45.20%	0.0057	8.232	636.05
DataStateCustomOverlap	23.73	3.50	44.96%	0.0864	18.671	19.45	4.23	3.41	35.59%	0.0496	5.710	20.58	263.53	9.44	39.36%	0.0060	6.898	636.05
ActivityWithBeforesAndData	46.31	1.12	89.71%	0.0133	0.312	1.38	19.87	1.85	60.73%	0.0298	1.855	5.79	364.24	4.28	56.84%	0.0046	136.28	136.71
ActivityWithBeforesAndDataAndCBs	25.64	1.13	89.62%	0.0155	0.420	1.42	6.96	1.79	63.85%	0.0291	1.549	5.41	361.76	2.85	60.00%	0.0044	1.941	31.34

scorer is not that far of the top performers. The latter even generally outperforms the activity similarity scorers on the EmergencyDepartment log. They have similar accuracy and brier scores, but RespondedFrequency scorer has a significantly better log loss and rank score. A closer analysis points the finger to the configuration of the similarity algorithm. We only used the 100 most similar traces from H to calculate the probability estimates of each potential next activity. Therefore, not all potential next activities are ranked for logs with close-to-or-more activities. If a scorer did not rank the correct next activity, we calculated its rank as the average ranking of all unranked recommendations. For example, the EmergencyDepartment log has 117 potential next activities (=116 activities + 1 end of trace). Suppose a scorer ranked 25 potential next activities, but the correct next activity was not among them. Then the rank of the correct next activity will be calculated as $25 + (117-25)/2 = 71$. Increasing the number of similar traces to consider could improve this, however, this would result in an increase in computation time.

The use of a data state similarity scorer to complement an activity similarity in the ActivityWithBeforesAndData scorer had mixed results. The combined scorer shows a slight improvement in the ArmFractures log compared to just the ActivityWithBefores scorer, but the results are opposite for the other two logs. We suspect that the chosen weights might have been the issue. The weight of the DataStateCustomOverlap similarity score is perhaps a too high (40%). This component has a slightly lower weight (32%), compared to its ActivityWithBefores component, in the slightly better performing ActivityWithBeforesAndDataAndKBs scorer. However, the increase in performance could also come from its RespondedFrequency component. Although, further experiments will be needed to draw any real conclusions about the complementary value of a data similarity scorer, the ActivityWithBeforesAndDataAndKBs scorer clearly combines the best of both worlds (RQ1). It has the predictive power of the similarity scorers and the consistency of the pre-calculated scorers for logs with a high number of activities. And finally, it is also worth noting that the computation time of the combined scorers typically is lower than the sum of the computation times of its component scorers. The explanation can be found in how the component similarity scorers are combined. They do not run in isolation, instead the combination of the similarity components is used directly in the variable-position algorithm. Thus, the convergence of this heuristic can differ from the convergence of the component scorers in isolation, albeit using an inherently slower similarity calculation.

5.2.6.2   Experiment 2: The Relation Between Predictive Power and the Size of H

5.2.6.2.1 Experimental Setup

In this experiment, we created sets containing a varying number of traces to serve as H and separate sets of traces to evaluate the scorers with. The two types of sets were randomly created and never contained overlapping traces. For each log, the size of the set of traces for evaluation was always the same for all sizes of H (500, 100 and 1657, respectively). The experiment ran 3 to 5 times for each size and the average over all runs was calculated. Otherwise, the setup and evaluation criteria were the same as in experiment 1.

5.2.6.2.2 Computational Results

The results of this experiment have been summarized in Fig. 5.31. The less interesting scorers (i.e., those that perform similar or worse than comparable strategies

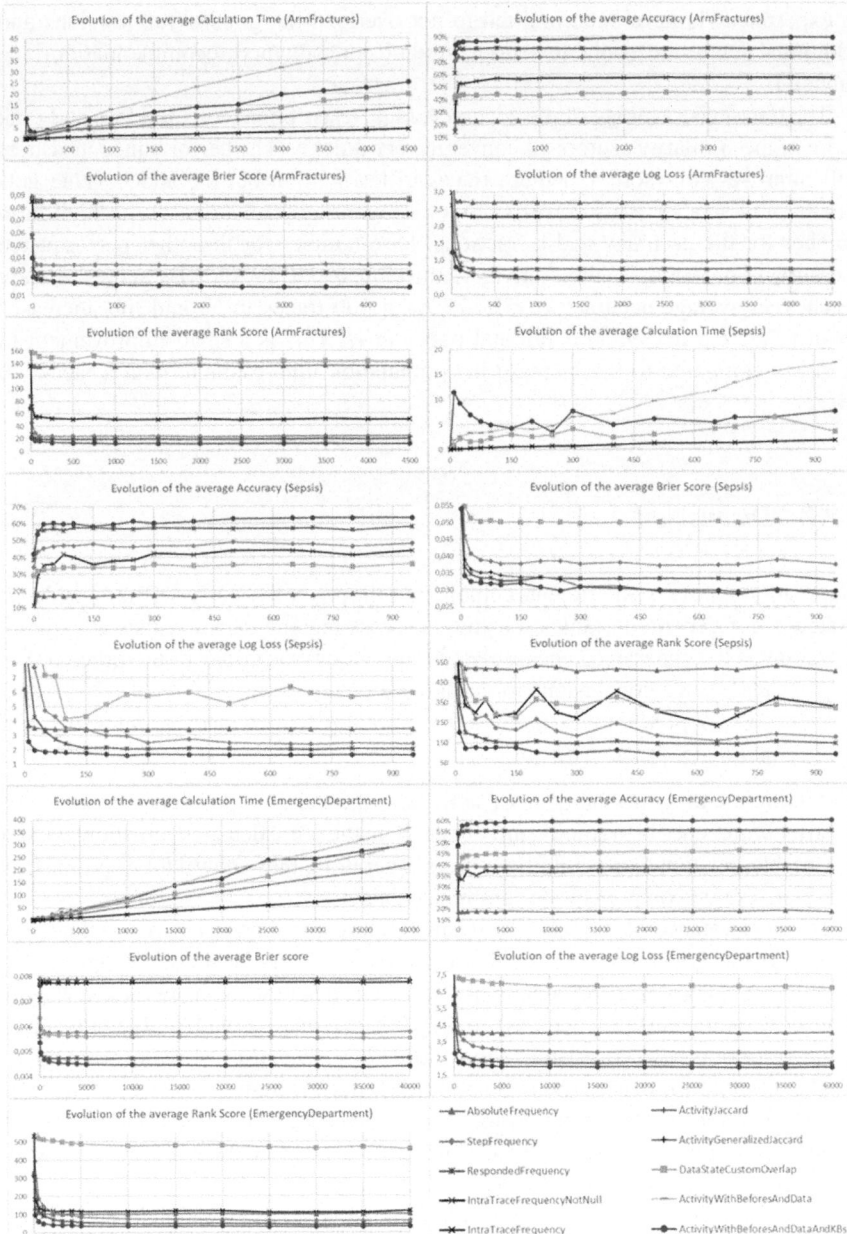

Fig. 5.2 The results for experiment 2

in experiment 1) have been omitted to not overload the graphs (full versions and additional details are available at https://github.com/stevmert/recommendationExpe riments).

The trace-wise average of the accuracy, multi-class brier score, log loss and rank score of the similarity scorers all converge very quickly. The performance measures still improve with more and more traces to learn from, but the added value gets smaller and smaller. This corresponds to a logarithmic relation: with a high base number for the accuracy and a fractional base number for the other performance measures. For example, the ActivityWithBeforesAndDataAndKBs scorer already reaches an average accuracy of 57.75% with 500 traces in H, and this increases by just 2.52% with 39500 additional traces in H. This is a small improvement in accuracy compared to the increase in computation time by more than a factor 40 (RQ3).

5.2.7 Discussion

The results of the two experiments demonstrate the predictive power of the considered strategies for generating ranked business process recommendation lists as a direct reflection of the experience encapsulated in previous executions of the process. We can formulate some conclusions for each research question.

RQ1: *Which prediction strategies perform well for knowledge-intensive and flexible healthcare* processes?

- For logs with a low number of activities, the variable-position activity simi- larity scorers perform significantly better than the pre-calculated, positionless and variable-position data similarity scorers. Therefore, they show a lot of promise as a high-weight component for combined strategies.
- The performance of the variable-position similarity scorers clearly declines for logs with a high number of activities, because of the limited number of ranked next activities. In this case, the penalty of a correct next activity being unranked weighs heavily on the performance. As we only had one data set with a high number of activities, it is hard to generalize this further or to even use a stricter formulation. The lower performance could also be attributed to the high complexity of the real- life EmergencyDepartement. Future experiments will determine if increasing the number of most similar traces to consider is a good countermeasure and what would be the corresponding impact on the computation times.
- The data and data state variable-position similarity scorers perform unsatisfactory across the board. This was expected, as we envisioned them to be more of an auxil- iary and low-weight component for combined scorers. The data state strategies show the most potential.
- Overall, the combined scorers come out on top for all performance measures. Only for the Sepsis log they are beaten by a few variable-position activity similarity scorers on the brier and rank scores, but we suspect this might be due to suboptimal

weights and a limited number of traces to learn from (i.e., 1050 compared to 5000 and 41657 for the other event logs). Choosing the subcomponents and weights more carefully, keeping in mind the experimental results from this work, could probably also get them to the top for the Sepsis log. Hyperparameter tuning algorithms can be applied to do this automatically.

- The Sepsis log was also used in Tax et al. [212], which compares several other next-element prediction strategies. As explained in Sect. 5.2.2, the goal of these predictions is a bit different to that of this work. However, the raw predictive power of the techniques can still be compared. Tax et al. use only the brier score to compare the performance of the techniques. Our best strategies outperform the baseline, process mining, machine learning compression, Markov and grammar inference techniques considered in that paper. The artificial neural network and all k-order Markov models (AKON) techniques did have better brier scores, but difference is small (0.0004 and 0.0019, respectively). Perhaps a more meticulous selection of subcomponents for a new combined scorer and some form of hyperparameter tuning would result in similar or even better brier scores. It is worth noting that a better brier score, although they are clearly correlated, does not necessarily mean that the other performance measures used in this work would agree. For example, the Activity scorer has a better average brier score for the Sepsis log in the first experiment, but a worse average rank, accuracy, log loss and rank score. Comparing the artificial neural network and all k-order Markov models (AKON) techniques using all of our performance measures on a more complex data set like the EmergencyDepartement log will hopefully provide a clearer picture in the future.

RQ2: *What kind of precision and consistency can be achieved and in what amount of computation time?*

- The achieved performance primarily depends on the characteristics of log. The variable-position activity similarity and combined scorers achieve an accuracy of almost 90% for the ArmFractures log, almost 64% for the Sepsis log and 60% for the EmergencyDepartment log. On average, the correct next activity will be in the top 2 of the variable-position activity similarity and combined scorers' recommendations for the ArmFractures and Sepsis logs, in the top 4 and top 3 for the variable-position activity similarity and combined scorers, respectively, for the EmergencyDepartment log. The rank scores for the ArmFractures and Sepsis logs show that the variable-position activity similarity scorers perform consistently for logs with relatively few unique activities, but when that number rises they tend to struggle a bit more. The precalculated scorers achieve better performance for the EmergencyDepartment log with its 116 unique activities, while the variable-position combined scorer that combines both takes the crown in consistency.
- The strong performance of the variable-position activity similarity and combined scorers does come at the expense of a higher average computation time. Where the pre-calculated scorers just need to retrieve the ranking from memory, the variable-position similarity scorers must calculate the similarity between the CPT and the

traces in H on the spot and subsequently analyze the most similar traces in H for what activity each has as next at its most similar position. However, even the highest average computation time is considerably less than one second. This certainly seems to be acceptable for real-life applications. Moreover, the results of the second experiment show that a relatively small size for H can offer almost the same performance, while severely reducing the computation time.

- The pre-calculated scorers have the lowest computation time, as expected, but even the relatively slow scorers only needed a little more than 0.6 s of computation time for even the biggest and most complex event log. This is an excellent result for these unoptimized implementations, albeit with more parallel processing power than might be typically available. It bodes well for its applicability in real-life settings, where a noticeably long computation time could be a source of frustration for the process actors using such a system.

RQ3: *How much data is needed to for near-optimal precision?*

Experiment 2 demonstrates that just a couple of hundred traces in H is sufficient for most cases concerning the datasets from this work or similar datasets. Large sizes for H are only sensible in situations where the maximal performance is required, and processing power is less of an issue. Of course, the exact number of traces required will strongly depend on the characteristics of process and the quality of the corresponding event log. Larger sizes of H could be needed to achieve near-optimal precision for processes with an even higher complexity or with datasets of lower quality.

RQ4: *Which strategies could be useful benchmarks to evaluate more advanced techniques (e.g., neural networks) in the future?*

The RespondedFrequency scorer, and to a lesser degree also the StepFrequency scorer, manages to consistently offer moderate-to-good performance, independent of the complexity and number of activities. The simplicity of the strategy and negligible computation time make it an easy-to-implement (or even fallback) option to provide some guidance. It can also be an excellent benchmark for more advanced strategies and techniques. The performance of the AbsoluteFrequency, ActivityInTraceFrequency, IntraTraceFrequency and IntraTraceFrequencyNotNull scorers is insufficient for these purposes. Their use should be limited to providing relative rankings for otherwise unranked or extremely unlikely next activities, as was the case for the ActivityWithBeforesAndDataAndKBs scorer.

5.2.8   Conclusion and Future Research

The results of the two experiments demonstrate the predictive power of the considered strategies when generating ranked process recommendation lists as a direct reflection of the experience encapsulated in previous executions of the process. Each strategy focuses on specific aspects of the process and they use all sorts of similarity metrics to relate partially executed traces to historic executions.

Although the results vary from log to log and even from performance measure to performance measure, some straightforward trends were revealed. Firstly, there are huge performance differences between the set of simple and pre-calculated strategies. The RespondedFrequency scorer is the clear-cut winner among this group of strategies with its consistent and moderate-to-good overall performance. This scorer seems like a great choice for a performance benchmark for more advanced techniques. Secondly, the variable-position activity similarity scorers unsurprisingly are top of the class of the scorers that focus on just one aspect of the process. Even for knowledge-intensive processes, previously executed activities seem like the best single-aspect predictors for the future activities, albeit with some meaningful differences between different strategies to represent the previously executed activities. Thirdly, the data and data state variable-position state similarity scorers can be useful as a component that complements another strategy, but not as a standalone scorer, and from this group of strategies, the data strategies that keep a data state are superior to those that do not. Fourthly, the drawbacks of single-aspect strategies can be mitigated by combining strategies. The results of the combined scorers demonstrate that combinations of strategies can outperform the separate building blocks, at a cost of a relatively small increase in computation time. Fifthly, the precision from the simple and unoptimized scorers used in this work is promising. For the ArmFractures log they could predict the correct next activity with an accuracy of just a hair under 90%. The two real-life logs were clearly more challenging as reflected by a maximal accuracy of 64% and 60%. However, this just reflects the number of times that the correct next activity was predicted as the first ranked recommendation. For offering guidance to the process actors it is still acceptable if the correct next activity was ranked near the top. The best performing scorers were able to rank the correct next activity on average in the top-2 or top-3 of their recommendations. This should ensure that the correct recommendation was at least within reasonable viewing range of the process actors. And finally, the computation time for the different strategies is manageable, even for complex real-life event logs. If necessary, the computation time can be reduced significantly by reducing the size of H (up to a small fraction of all available data) with relatively minimal impact on the overall performance of the scorer.

As part of the future research, we plan to investigate the impact of increasing the number of similar traces used in the variable-position similarity scorers and the use of trace encodings to improve memory usage. For the scorers themselves, we will consider optimizations, hyperparameter tuning and more combinations of strategies. Advanced techniques like neural networks will also be considered and compared. At a more general level, we would like to apply the techniques to many more event logs. The idea is that this might reveal preferred strategies or techniques for processes on different parts of the flexibility and/or knowledge-intensity spectrum.

Research Contributions of Chapter 5

- A generic framework for creating data-aware declarative BPEs
- The proof-of-concept tool support of the framework: DeciClareEngine

- A set of 40 next-activity prediction strategies that can be used as the foundation for a process recommendation generator
- The prediction strategies that perform well for loosely framed KiPs (excluding black-box techniques)
- An idea of the precision and consistency can be achieved by the prediction strategies in a certain amount of computation time
- The amount of data that is required by the prediction strategies for near-optimal precision
- The prediction strategies that could be useful benchmarks to evaluate other strategies, black-box strategies (e.g., neural networks) in particular, in the future

Chapter 6
Conclusion and Future Research

6.1 Research Results

The starting point of this dissertation was the observation that current BPM techniques and corresponding BPMSs are not well suited for managing and supporting loosely framed KiPs. They have problems with the complexity that arises from both the loosely framed and knowledge-intensive character of these processes. The result is a very limited adoption of BPM in sectors were KiPs are common (e.g., healthcare, legal profession etc.). Section 1.3 listed three specific objectives that form the foundation of a BPMS for loosely framed KiPs, the development of which was the general objective of this dissertation. The resulting research contributions for each of these objectives, are summarized below.

Objective 1: The development of a declarative process modeling language that suits loosely framed KiPs, which lays the foundation for the Process Designer-component of the BPMS.

- A feature analysis of existing declarative process (Declare, Timed Declare, TBDeclare, ConDec-R, Data-aware Declare, Declare++ and Declare based on LTL-FO) and decision (DMN) modeling languages
- Metamodels of existing declarative languages (Declare and ConDec-R)
- The DeciClare declarative process and decision modeling language, with integrated functional, control-flow, data and resource perspectives
- The DeciClare Process Designer-component (textual)

The core problem is a mismatch between the characteristics of loosely framed KiPs and the leading modeling paradigm, which takes on an imperative viewpoint. The imperative modeling paradigm thrives in settings with little variation but degenerates to useless spaghetti models in settings were executional flexibility is crucial. The stakeholders of loosely framed processes are left with the impossible choice to either artificially reduce the executional freedom they need to operate properly in order to

© Springer Nature Switzerland AG 2020
S. Mertens: Enabling Process Management for Loosely Framed
Knowledge-Intensive Processes, LNBIP 409,
https://doi.org/10.1007/978-3-030-66193-9_6

accommodate mainstream BPM techniques, or just reject the adoption of most of these techniques and perpetuate the current overextension of knowledge workers that lacks transparency and often also efficiency. Therefore, a paradigm shift is essential to provide them with the process support they need. The declarative modeling paradigm has been proposed before as a potential solution. It offers flexibility by design, without the requirement to enumerate every possible valid process variation explicitly. With the addition of resource and data perspectives, a declarative modeling language can also cater to the knowledge-intensive characteristics. The former is needed to model the multidisciplinary aspects of many knowledge-intensive processes, while the latter enables modeling the decisions that govern the choice for a specific process variation. The disadvantage of the declarative paradigm compared to imperative paradigm comes down to human understandability. Declarative models have less or even no explicit flow, and therefore are inherently difficult for humans to comprehend easily. Declarative languages like DCR Graphs try to mitigate this problem by limiting the number of constraint types and providing a clear visual syntax. However, in the scope of this dissertation, the models are targeted more towards automated interpretation by computers, and so, this disadvantage is less relevant.

For the fulfillment of the objective, we first listed the requirements for a modeling language for loosely framed KiPs. Based on these requirements, we analyzed the features of existing declarative process modeling languages. The DeciClare modeling language was subsequently developed by incorporating features of the existing languages and several new features to satisfy the requirements. The domain appropriateness was evaluated by domain experts to verify a good match between the characteristics of loosely framed KiPs and the newly developed modeling language.

Objective 2: The development of a method for process and decision discovery of loosely framed KiPs for the Process Discovery-component of the BPMS, and a corresponding mining technique that can mine a process and decision model from an event log.

- The DeciClareMiner process and decision mining technique and corresponding tool
- A method for process and decision discovery of loosely framed KiPs for the Process Discovery-component that uses the DeciClareMiner process mining technique
- A case study evaluation at the emergency medicine department of AZ Maria Middelares, Ghent, Belgium

Process discovery is traditionally done by way of interviews with process actors and other domain experts. This is straightforward when there is little knowledge to extract, but otherwise can quickly become a very difficult, effort-intensive, time-consuming and error-prone task for both the modeler and the process actors. The manual discovery of loosely framed KiPs certainly falls in the latter category. Most of the process knowledge is tacit and scattered over the multi-disciplinary team of process actors. Process mining techniques offers an alternative way of extracting some of this knowledge, if enough digital process data is available and that data is of sufficient quality. Therefore, we developed a process and decision mining technique, DeciClareMiner, that can discover a model written in the declarative modeling language that was the result of objective 1. It consists of two phases. The first phase consists of a complete search algorithm inspired by the Apriori association rule mining algorithm, while the second phase uses a heuristic belonging to the class of genetic algorithms. This difference in approach for each phase is rooted in the assumption that in the context of loosely framed KiPs, the number of possible activities will be much lower than the number of combinations of available data elements on which decisions are based. This means that using a complete-search algorithm for the first phase is acceptable, while for the second phase, a heuristic is more appropriate. Additionally, the search space of the second phase algorithm was significantly reduced by efficiently making use of a subset of constraints that was discarded, but stored, during the first phase (i.e., minimal rules). The output is a model of the process that describes the given process both in terms of the process control-flow and the decisions that govern the control-flow.

The literature on process mining often assumes that a satisfactory event log is available, and that the execution of the process mining technique is the only step of a discovery project. However, this is not a good reflection of reality. The process mining techniques are just part of one step of a more general method to discover processes. Two methodologies to perform process discovery have been published, but they presume the use of an imperative process mining technique. So, a new method was developed that consists of gathering the necessary data, structuring that data, preparing the resulting event log, mining a declarative model and evaluating that model. These steps should be repeated iteratively until a satisfactory model is discovered. Of course, the method centers around the use of the DeciClareMiner technique, but the quality of the output dependents at least as much on the other steps, if not more, due to importance of data quantity and quality. During the development of the method, we simultaneously applied it to real data from the emergency care process that takes place in the medical emergency department of a hospital. The result was a process and decision model that successfully transformed some of the tacit process knowledge to explicit knowledge. Instead of numerous and time-consuming interviews with the process actors, it merely required an occasional interview with one domain expert to evaluate the discovered model for each iteration.

Objective 3: The development of a BPE- and Process Analytics-component for the BPMS that can offer support and guidance to the process actors during process execution.

- The DeciClare BPE-component that supports

  - Process execution
  - Runtime conformance checking
  - Process replay capabilities

- A recommendation generator for the BPE-component that provides guidance to the users and is the first part of the Process Analytics-component

The development of a process and decision modeling language and mining technique for loosely framed KiPs fulfills the first two objectives. The declarative paradigm of the resulting models represents many process variations implicitly, which is good for modeling and discovery but difficult for humans to interpret due to the lack of explicit process paths to follow. Computers are much better at interpreting declarative models. Therefore, an automated system to support users that need to execute a declarative model would be very helpful. This is typically a job for a BPMS, and more specifically, the BPE-component of a BPMS. A BPE automatically interprets a given model and presents the user only with the actions that are allowed by the model in the current phase of the execution of a process instance. Traditional BPEs execute imperative process models that often consist of just one or two explicit process paths. They are not capable of executing a declarative process model, hence, a new type of BPE needed to be developed. Additionally, the new BPE also needed to be able to handle the extensive data perspective of the declarative process and decision modeling language that resulted from objective 1. The problem was tackled by creating a BPE that categorizes the activities according to whether or not they are allowed as next activity by the given model in the current context of the running process instance at hand both from a control-flow and data perspective. The users must then merely decide between the activities that are allowed by the model, keeping in mind any potential consequences that are noted by the engine (e.g., an additional activity must to be executed at a later time). The reasons why other activities are prohibited by the model are also provided so that the users can better understand the calculated categorization of activities. The result is that users are relieved of the difficult task of interpreting the model and can focus their full attention on the decision-making tasks, for which they are presented with all information available in the given model. However, as the processes are highly flexible, the model will often allow multiple activities to be performed next. Therefore, we investigated ways to provide additional guidance on which of the available next activities are preferable or typical in the current context of the running instance. A solution was devised that ranks the available next activities as process recommendations based on their frequency of occurring as the next activity in the most similar previously completed process instances. The rank and probability estimation of the process recommendations convey to the users how current and past knowledge workers of the organization would proceed, and hence, offer a direct reflection of the combined past and present experience in the organization. Many strategies from related literature to implement this type of recommendation generator, complemented with some novel strategies, were evaluated and compared. Eventually, this recommendation generator will be part of the Process Analytics component of the BPMS for loosely frame KiPs, along with other algorithms for different analytics tasks.

6.2 Research Relevance and Implications

Although many loosely framed KiPs are an integral part of our daily life, the process management support for these types of processes is severely lacking. In this dissertation we developed the fundamental building blocks needed to provide a basic level of process management, similar to how this is already available for other types of processes. The implication of the dissertation can be divided along two interest groups: researchers and process stakeholders.

6.2.1 Implications for Researchers

First off, the developed components for a BPMS for loosely framed KiPs can be the foundation for new decision support system research, as alternative to current lines of research into guidelines implementation and expert systems. The application of BPM in this context has not yet been thoroughly researched, both from a theoretical and empirical viewpoint. Secondly, new process monitoring, conformance-checking and simulation research avenues can be explored due to the higher expressive power of the developed process modeling language compared to previously available languages. And finally, a lot of research has now been enabled towards finding the best ways to incorporate these systems and techniques into practice. The foundation for the technical side has been provided, but the adoption of the resulting systems and techniques in practice requires more research into when, what and how to present them to the process stakeholders.

6.2.2 Implications for Process Stakeholders

The managers and other stakeholders of loosely framed KiPs are now often left in the dark about what is happening and why. The results of this dissertation can be used to transform a lot the tacit knowledge and experience into explicit knowledge that can be analyzed to gain valuable insight into these processes. The implication of this are plentiful:

- Knowledge workers are relieved of some of the more time-consuming task of having to reinvent the wheel over an over to determine a path towards a satisfactory process ending. They get the necessary support for applying all the rules, guidelines and norms of the organization and can fully focus on the execution of the actual process activities and the crucial decision-making tasks along the way.
- Having explicit rules for the occurrence and sequencing of activities and the corresponding decision logic enables available deeper analysis and optimization of the working habits of knowledge workers. The decision logic in the models can also be compared to the available guidelines (e.g., Are the guidelines properly applied? If not, what are the characteristic and decision criteria of the cases in which they diverge from the guidelines? Are these justifiable?).

- The explicit knowledge extracted by the proposed techniques can be used as an explicit justification as to why certain activities are performed in specific cases and others are not.
- The service offered as a result of the execution of the loosely framed KiPs can potentially be made to be more uniform. The current lack of transparency and support makes it difficult for the knowledge workers to gage how their own habits compare to those of their colleagues. By making the process more transparent and providing insight to how the knowledge workers' habits stack up to those of their colleagues, we would assume that this would lead to a more uniform way of executing the process.
- The mined models can be used for evidence farming [147]. This is the practice of posteriori analysis of data to find new insights without setting up case-control studies. Evidence farming can be used as an alternative or, even better, as a supplement to evidence-based knowledge gathering.
- New findings and working habits can be communicated and enforced directly though the BPMS by adding them to the process model.
- Every organization must deal with employee churn, but for loosely framed KiPs it can be even more devastating. An experienced knowledge worker cannot be replaced easily, and his/her knowledge and experience are typically lost. Even when an experienced replacement can be found, there is no way to tell if the replacement adequately compensates the loss. The proposed BPMS can make sure that not all of the knowledge and experience of the departing employee is lost, because some of the knowledge and all of the experiences and tendencies of the departing employee during his/her stay at the organization were captured in the data of the system. The knowledge captured in the data will have been made explicit in the model used by the BPMS and the experiences and tendencies have been made available through the recommendation generator. This makes the loss a bit less devastating, because the models can be used to educate new employees. Additionally, the experiences and tendencies of current and past colleagues made available by the recommendation generator will provide the necessary support to bring them up to speed more quickly.
- The educational value for new employees can also be generalized to improve educational system that supplies future knowledge workers. The models and recommendations could be used in direct teaching methods, but also to provide realistic replay and simulation capabilities that better prepare them for the job and support them when they are eventually deployed.

Many of the above implications require the input data for the discovery and recommendations to reach a certain level of data quality and detail. For the former we can also make a distinction between the level of detail of the activity definitions (e.g., 'request lab-tests' vs. 'request urine test for nickel poising') and of the contextual data ('pain' vs. 'pain in shoulder' vs. 'pain in shoulder when moving the arm upwards'), while the latter relates to all data in general. The required levels are hard to quantify, as they depend on the use case and inherent complexity of the underlying process. The more complex the patterns and decisions that need to be identified, the higher the levels of data quality and detail that must be achieved. In my opinion, the data quality and level of detail in the activity definitions should be prioritized over the level of detail of the contextual data, because the data quality directly relates to the confidence one should have in the applications and the activity definitions directly relates to the type of knowledge that can be made explicit. These both heavily influence the usefulness, user-friendliness and amount of guidance any the applications can offer.

On the flip side, increasing the level of detail in the input data will incur a cost computationally: the search space that the process mining tool must cover increases exponentially as it grows, the BPE will be slower to categorize the potential next activities due to more complex models and the recommendations generator will be slower to provide recommendations and predictions due to more data needing to be compared. Therefore, this important tradeoff between speed and precision must certainly be carefully considered. Note that increasing the data quality does not necessarily come at a computational cost. This is another reason to prioritize the data quality in these kinds of projects.

6.2.3 Generalizability to Other Domains

This dissertation focusses heavily on the healthcare domain, because it is perhaps the most extreme example, but loosely framed KiPs occur in many other branches of the service industry. Consider the following examples:

- Legal profession: liability lawyers are hired by individuals or companies to represent them in a legal battle over liability in some event. After reviewing the case at hand and speaking with the client, they must establish a legal strategy by making an interpretation of the law. Based on the strategy they go into a negotiation with the legal teams of the other parties in the case, request evidence to be turned over, review evidence, request different types of expert testimony, search for legal precedent, etc. Additionally, they must respect the procedural rules of the specific court in front of which they are to appear (i.e., timely send documents, requests and notifications to court officials and other parties). If no agreement was reached, the case goes to trial. During the trial, all parties plead their cases to a judge, who will eventually hand out a verdict. A verdict does not necessarily mean the end of the case, as any one of the involved parties could decide to fight the decision based on the available grounds for appeal of the specific court that gave the verdict. This could start a new round in the legal battle with different procedures depending on the new court to which the case would be moved.
  In comparison with the healthcare cases from this dissertation, the activities before a trial are comparable to diagnostic tests, a verdict to a preliminary diagnosis and an appeal to a preliminary diagnosis turning out to be wrong. A trial is more like surgery, because what goes on during is beyond the scope of the system proposed in this dissertation. Therefore, it should be treated like an atomic activity. The

abundance of legal strategies, procedures, interpretations of the law and legal precedents leads to much variation and scattered knowledge, while the execution of the process depends heavily decisions made by the lawyers involved based their knowledge and experience.

- Customer services: customer service agents are contacted by customers with a complaint. The subject of a case can be just about anything related to the products or services offered by the company for which the they provide customer service. The customer service agent must first gather information about the problem by listening to the customer and asking the right questions. With this information, the agent can start examining the problem and possibly order internal investigations of the malfunctioning product or service. Based on the findings, the agent can consider different ways to resolve the problem or at least appease the customer. The agent might also have to ask permission from his/her manager for some of the resolution options.

  The job of a customer service agent shows a lot of similarity to the healthcare examples presented in this dissertation. They also must diagnose a problem based on the symptoms as described by the customer, investigate the problem with diagnostic tests or support from the experts from within the company, and propose solutions to resolve the problems (i.e., a treatment). The difference mostly relates to the level of flexibility and decision autonomy permitted to the customer service agents. Their decision autonomy and options available for investigation and resolution are often limited in real-life, arguably to the detriment of all stakeholders (i.e., less satisfied customers lead to reputation damage and lost revenue for the company). In my own experience, smaller companies often permit their agents more decision autonomy, which they use to provide a better and more personalized service.

- Air traffic control: air traffic controllers are responsible for safe and efficient incoming, outgoing and overflying air traffic in a controlled airspace. They must communicate with pilots, airport personnel and other air traffic controllers, manage the four-dimensional movement of the air traffic, constantly determine the priority of events, make safety adjustments were needed and deal with all sorts of emergency situations.

  Although it is harder to draw a direct parallel with the healthcare cases of this dissertation, this is certainly a loosely framed KiP. The controller must constantly use his/her knowledge and experience to maintain an overview of the situation, assess threats, make split-second decisions and intervene timely when necessary, while the unique context of each situation and the multitude of other actors and possible actions results in a high need for run-time flexibility.

Each of these examples display the characteristics of loosely framed KiPs and the same external pressure to provide more service in less time. The differences between these other examples and the healthcare cases used throughout this dissertation relate predominantly to the interactions with the clients and how stationary that the knowledge workers are during the execution of these processes. Lawyer often have with little contact with their clients, just enough to keep them up-to-date. Customer service agents and air traffic controllers, in contrast, are in constant audio communication with their clients (i.e., customers and pilots, respectively). And while physicians are typically running around and having direct contact with the clients (i.e., patients), lawyers, customer service agents and air traffic controllers generally do most of their work on their computer at their desk. The fact that the knowledge workers in these other domains are mostly stationary, should make it easier to capture the process execution data. For customer service agents and air traffic controllers this is certainly the case, while lawyers are starting to catch up by utilizing more and more digital technology. And so, the benefits of the system proposed in this dissertation should also hold true for other domains that house loosely framed KiPs.

6.2.4 Research Limitations and Future Research

In this dissertation, several proof-of-concept tools and techniques were proposed. A proof-of-concept demonstrates the core principles of a design artifact. Therefore, it does not require every feature or aspect that might be needed for general usage. The missing features and aspects of the proposed artifacts are listed below, as well as some additionally interesting avenues for future research.

- The DeciClare process modeling languages has an expressive metamodel and corresponding set of constraint templates. However, the current visualization is merely textual. A real visual syntax is yet to be developed and could potentially make it easier for users to quickly understand a model or parts of it.
- The DeciClareMiner process discovery technique can already handle the 9 most frequently used templates (out of 36). However, the support will be further expanded. Additionally, the feasibility of mining information and resources templates from process data will to be investigated. This will require some resource-related data that is not yet available in common event logs, but perhaps the logs can be enriched with this data.
- The models that DeciClareMiner returns when the confidence is set to less than 100% can contain inconsistencies. This is because a rule that conforms to 90 out of 100 instances in which it is activated (e.g., do activity 1 next), can be inconsistent with a rule that conforms perfectly (or at least more than the confor-mance threshold) to the 10 missing instances (e.g., do activity 2 next). For these 10 instances, the model will demand two contradictory actions. Techniques to resolve issues like this have been proposed for Declare [175], but they will need to be adapted to become useful for DeciClare due to its support for (de-) activation decisions.
- The inclusion of more advanced text mining and natural language processing techniques, like TiMBL, in the 'Log preparation'-step of the method for process and decision discovery of loosely framed KiPs will be further investigated. This has the potential to improve the data quality of the resulting event log, which in turn can improve the discovered process and decision models.

- The BPE-component, DeciClareEngine, already supports 17 of the 36 constraint templates of DeciClare, but the support is not yet complete. Support for the remaining templates will be added in the future, as well as for deactivation decisions. However, not all of these templates can be enforced by a BPE (e.g., 'at least 5 nurses need to be available'). Additionally, methods for partial live- or deadlock detection or prevention will be investigated. At a practical level, support will also be added for dynamic resource availabilities and parallel execution of activities, while more efficient validation techniques will be investigated to speed up the engine. And finally, more advanced simulation capabilities will be added to the engine on top of the current replay capabilities of historic instances.
- The current recommendation generator only makes suggestions for the next activity to be executed. We will investigate whether it would be beneficial to also include sequences of multiple activities to be executed next. This could be because of standard procedure, as part of a medical guideline or just because the choice for the first activity of the sequence predetermines the others. This has the potential to make of the consequences of a decision more explicit. Those consequences will also be made clearer by providing the user with an overview of the differences in the impact of each recommendation on the remainder the current instance (e.g., activity X is prohibited in case recommendation 1 is selected but selecting recommendation 2 would mean activity X is available afterwards).
- The techniques behind the recommendation generator can also be used to provide the user with predictions of key performance indicators (KPIs) and other process characteristics (e.g., remaining time, urgency cost, etc.). This predictive component will become the process analytics component of the BPMS for loosely framed KiPs.
- The decision modeling aspect of DeciClare focusses on the specific combinations of data values that lead to certain behavior (e.g., if a patient has a suspected lower arm fracture then a scan needs to be made), but these data values are just the consequences of an actual decision rationale that was applied (e.g., a scan is needed to check if there is indeed a fracture and, if so to determine the position of the fractured bone endings). The decision rationale is certainly more valuable knowledge. During the first stages of this research project, it quickly became clear that we lacked the means to make the decision rationales explicit without requiring a huge time and effort investment of the knowledge workers. The only options to gather some data on decision rationales are through interviews or by asking the knowledge workers to think aloud during their daily tasks and recording this. The former is often inefficient and incomplete, while the latter is very invasive and difficult to use on a large scale. So, we focused on the data that was already being captured (i.e., the process data in the information systems of an organization). However, this data is not sufficiently rich to reconstruct the decision rationales. The quality of a system as envisioned in this dissertation could certainly benefit if users would be motivated to include the rationale in the data, as complementary data, so future work should certainly explore this path.

Appendix A: Arm Fracture Case Description (Based on Literature)

The process of treating arm-related fractures takes place in the emergency and orthopedic department of a hospital. The process entails the registration, diagnosis and treatment phases for patients with suspected fractures of a finger, hand, wrist, forearm, upper arm, shoulder, and/or collarbone.

The process starts when a patient is registered at the reception of the emergency department. Alternatively, in acute emergency situations, the registration can be done at a later time. The next step will usually be to take a medical history (e.g., previous injuries and medication) and perform a clinical examination of the patient. During this the doctor will make enquiries as to the current symptoms (e.g., excessive pain and deformation) of the patient and perform a hands-on examination. Based on these symptoms the doctor will make a preliminary diagnosis. Normally, this diagnosis is checked by making X-rays, which in turn always results in a new doctor-patient consultation to evaluate the X-rays and make the actual diagnosis. In some situations, the doctor can make the final diagnosis without X-rays (e.g., clearly no fracture). In some cases, a complementary CT-scan will be used to get even more information.

The next phase involves the treatment the patient will receive. Of course, a treatment is only possible after a preliminary clinical examination by a doctor. There are 9 possible treatments: prescribing rest (= no treatment), applying ice, managing pain with pain medication, applying a bandage, applying a splint, providing support with a sling, fixating the fracture, applying a cast or performing surgery. Choosing one does not eliminate other treatments, as some treatment strategies combine two or more treatments. It is also possible that ice, a sling, some bandages and/or a splint is applied at any time during the process in order to make the patient as comfortable as possible, no matter the diagnosis.

When we look at the case on a more detailed level we can identify several different variations. These represent the classes of fractures that can occur. Each has a specific flow and different characteristics to be taken into account. One common characteristic is that all fractures require surgery if the fracture is open or displaced. Also, if there is no emergency situation, a fracture diagnosis will need to be confirmed by an X-ray (usually also in emergency situations depending on the type of injury).

- A fractured finger or a fractured bone in his hand: in most cases a simple fixation is enough to let it heal. The patient will receive a sling before being sent home.
- A fractured wrist: a cast will be applied, possibly after performing surgery. Surgery is required if the patient is a child (less than 15 years old) and has a damaged periosteum. For adults, surgery is only performed when dealing with open or complex fractures. Afterwards a follow-up X-ray will be taken to confirm that the bone is positioned correctly to start the healing process. The patient will receive a sling be-fore being sent home.

- A fractured forearm: usually this requires no more than a cast. Only when the bone parts are too far apart, surgery is required. To support the cast, the patient receives a sling before being sent home.
- A fractured upper arm: is commonly treated by applying a fixation. The patient will receive a sling before being sent home.
- A fractured shoulder: usually the conservative treatment is enough, letting the shoulder heal while wearing a sling. In the other cases, surgery is required. Physio-therapy is also needed, because the shoulder joint will be inactive for an extended period during either of both treatments.
- A fractured collarbone: is treated in most cases by resting it while wearing a figure of eight bandage. Surgery is only required when dealing with open or complex fractures or extensive damage to the arteries or nerves.

Additionally, if surgery is required for a broken wrist or forearm, but the OR is unavailable, a temporary cast will be applied to bridge the time until surgery can be performed.

Another aspect is the prescription of medication. There is a general policy that states that no medication can be prescribed without being preceded by an actual doctor's examination. For pain medication it also requires the doctor or surgeon to agree that the patient is in pain or could be in pain in the nearby future. After surgery patients will be prescribed anticoagulants and a painkiller as precaution. In many cases an additional stomach protecting drug is given to counteract possible detrimental side effects of the other two prescriptions. Furthermore, patients that received a cast could be prescribed anticoagulants. Because there exist strong painkillers that do not mix well with anti-coagulants, a distinction is made between classes of painkillers:

- Painkillers A: should not be taken while on anticoagulants but are preferred in other cases.
- Painkillers B: can be taken while on anticoagulants.

We also need to consider that some activities require the availability of certain resources, which in turn are limited in number. Also, they are not only used for this process, but rather represent a pool of resources shared among multiple independent processes of the hospital. The inventory of the material resources as used during the process goes as follows:

- Reception desks
- Exam rooms
- X-ray rooms with an X-ray machine
- CT-scan room with an CT-scanner
- Operating rooms
- Recovery room beds
- Patient rooms
- Patient beds
- Physiotherapy room
- Furthermore, there is also a list of human resources available:
- Receptionists
- Nurses

- Doctors
  - Anesthesiologist
  - Orthopedic surgeon
  - Emergency doctors

- Surgical assistant
- Physiotherapist
- Some of the assumptions made:
- Patients do not go home until the process instance in finished
- Other medical issues are out of scope
- Patients do not refuse the recommended treatments

Appendix B: Original Textual DeciClare Model of Arm Fracture Case

Available Resources

[nurse, doctor, receptionist, surgeon, physiotherapist, reception desk, examination room, x-ray room, operating room, patient bed, physiotherapy room]

Available Activities

[Register patient, Examine patient, Take X-ray, Prescribe weak painkillers, Prescribe strong painkillers A, Prescribe strong painkillers B, Prescribe anticoagulants, Prescribe anti-inflammatory drugs, Apply cast, Apply sling, Apply fixation, Apply bandage, Apply figure of eight bandage, Perform surgery, Let patient rest, Perform physiotherapy]

Available Data Elements

[Clear emergency? = (True/False), Where there complications during surgery? = (True/False), Open or complex fracture? = (True/False), Extensive damage to arteries or nerves? = (True/False), Both arms broken? = (True/False), No improvement in 3 months? = (True/False), More than 16yrs old? = (True/False), Periosteum torn? = (True/False), OR available? = (True/False), Bone parts far apart? = (True/False), In pain (now or in foreseeable future)? = (True/False), On weak painkillers? = (True/False), On anticoagulants? = (True/False), On anti-inflammatory drugs? = (True/False), Fractured bone? = (Wrist/Forearm/Shoulder/Finger/Upper arm/Hand/Collarbone)]

Resource Constraints

- there are 10 nurses available
- there are 3 doctors available
- there are 2 receptionists available
- there are 2 surgeons available
- there is 1 physiotherapist available
- there are 2 reception desks available
- there are 15 examination rooms available
- there are 3 operating rooms available
- there is 1 x-ray room available
- there are 60 patient beds available
- there is 1 physiotherapy room available
- the execution of activity 'Register patient' requires a 'reception desk'
- the execution of activity 'Register patient' requires a 'receptionist'
- *If[['Clear emergency? = false']] then*
  the execution of activity 'Examine patient' requires an 'examination room'
- the execution of activity 'Examine patient' requires a 'doctor'

- the execution of activity 'Take X-ray' requires a 'x-ray room'
- the execution of activity 'Take X-ray' requires a 'doctor' or 'nurse'
- the execution of activity 'Apply cast' requires an 'examination room'
- the execution of activity 'Apply cast' requires a 'doctor' or 'nurse'
- the execution of activity 'Apply fixation' requires an 'examination room'
- the execution of activity 'Apply fixation' requires a 'doctor' or 'nurse'
- the execution of activity 'Apply figure of eight bandage' requires an 'examination room'
- the execution of activity 'Apply figure of eight bandage' requires a 'doctor' or 'nurse'
- the execution of activity 'Apply bandage' requires an 'examination room'
- the execution of activity 'Apply bandage' requires a 'doctor' or 'nurse'
- the execution of activity 'Apply sling' requires an 'examination room'
- the execution of activity 'Apply sling' requires a 'doctor' or 'nurse'
- the execution of activity 'Perform surgery' requires an 'operating room'
- the execution of activity 'Perform surgery' requires a 'surgeon'
- the execution of activity 'Let patient rest' requires a 'patient bed'
- the execution of activity 'Perform physiotherapy' requires a 'physiotherapy room'
- the execution of activity 'Perform physiotherapy' requires a 'physiotherapist'
- the execution of activity 'Prescribe weak painkillers' requires a 'doctor'
- the execution of activity 'Prescribe strong painkillers A' requires a 'doctor'
- the execution of activity 'Prescribe strong painkillers B' requires a 'doctor'
- the execution of activity 'Prescribe anticoagulants' requires a 'doctor'
- the execution of activity 'Prescribe anti-inflammatory drugs' requires a 'doctor'

Control-Flow Constraints

- *If[['Clear emergency? = false']] then*
  'Register patient' has to be performed as the first activity
- 'Register patient' has to be performed at least 1 time
- 'Register patient' can be performed at most 1 time
- 'Examine patient' has to be performed at least 1 time
- 'Apply sling' can be performed at most 2 times
- at least 1 out of 6 of the following activities have to be performed: 'Apply sling', 'Apply figure of eight bandage', 'Apply fixation', 'Apply cast', 'Perform surgery' and 'Apply bandage'
- *If[['Clear emergency? = false']] then*
- 'Register patient' has to precede 'Examine patient'
- 'Examine patient' has to precede 'Take X-ray'
- 'Take X-ray' has to be followed by 'Examine patient'
- 'Examine patient' has to precede 'Prescribe weak painkillers'
- 'Examine patient' has to precede 'Prescribe strong painkillers A'
- 'Examine patient' has to precede 'Prescribe strong painkillers B'
- 'Examine patient' has to precede 'Prescribe anticoagulants'
- 'Examine patient' has to precede 'Perform surgery'

- 'Examine patient' has to precede 'Apply fixation'
- 'Examine patient' has to precede 'Apply cast'
- 'Examine patient' has to precede 'Apply figure of eight bandage'
- 'Prescribe strong painkillers A' cannot be followed by 'Prescribe anticoagulants' within at most 5 days
- 'Prescribe anticoagulants' cannot be followed by 'Prescribe strong painkillers A' within at most 5 days
- *If[['Where there complications during surgery? = false']] then* 'Perform surgery' has to be followed by 'Let patient rest' within at most 5 min
- *If[['Open or complex fracture? = false' and 'Fractured bone? = Upper arm' and 'Extensive damage to arteries or nerves? = false' and 'Both arms broken? = false' and 'No improvement in 3 months? = false'] or ['Open or complex fracture? = false' and 'Fractured bone? = Hand' and 'Extensive damage to arteries or nerves? = false'] or ['Open or complex fracture? = false' and 'Fractured bone? = Finger' and 'Extensive damage to arteries or nerves? = false']] then* 'Apply fixation' has to be performed at least 1 time
- *If[['Open or complex fracture? = false' and 'Fractured bone? = Forearm' and 'Extensive damage to arteries or nerves? = false'] or ['Open or complex fracture? = false' and 'Extensive damage to arteries or nerves? = false' and 'More than 16yrs old? = false' and 'Fractured bone? = Wrist' and 'Periosteum torn? = false'] or ['Open or complex fracture? = false' and 'Extensive damage to arteries or nerves? = false' and 'Fractured bone? = Wrist' and 'More than 16yrs old? = true'] or ['Open or complex fracture? = false' and 'Fractured bone? = Shoulder' and 'Extensive damage to arteries or nerves? = false']] then* 'Apply cast' has to be performed at least 1 time
- *If[['Extensive damage to arteries or nerves? = true' and 'Fractured bone? = Forearm' and 'OR available? = false'] or ['Extensive damage to arteries or nerves? = true' and 'Fractured bone? = Wrist' and 'OR available? = false'] or ['Open or complex fracture? = true' and 'Fractured bone? = Wrist' and 'OR available? = false'] or ['Fractured bone? = Forearm' and 'Open or complex fracture? = true' and 'OR available? = false']] then* 'Apply cast' has to be performed at least 2 times
- *If[['Open or complex fracture? = false' and 'Extensive damage to arteries or nerves? = false' and 'Fractured bone? = Collarbone']] then* 'Apply figure of eight bandage' has to be performed at least 1 time
- *If[['Open or complex fracture? = false' and 'Periosteum torn? = true' and 'Extensive damage to arteries or nerves? = false' and 'More than 16yrs old? = false' and 'Fractured bone? = Wrist'] or ['Extensive damage to arteries or nerves? = true'] or ['Open or complex fracture? = false' and 'No improvement in 3 months? = true' and 'Fractured bone? = Upper arm' and 'Extensive damage to arteries or nerves? = false'] or ['Extensive damage to arteries or nerves? = true' and 'Fractured bone? = Forearm' and 'OR available? = false'] or ['Open or complex fracture? = true'] or ['Extensive damage to arteries or nerves? = true' and 'Fractured bone? = Wrist' and 'OR available? = false'] or ['Open or complex fracture? = false' and 'Fractured bone? = Upper arm' and 'Extensive damage to arteries or nerves? = false' and 'Both arms broken? = true']] then*

'Perform surgery' has to be performed at least 1 time

- *If[['Fractured bone? = Forearm' and 'Open or complex fracture? = true'] or ['Open or complex fracture? = true' and 'Fractured bone? = Wrist'] or ['Extensive damage to arteries or nerves? = true' and 'Fractured bone? = Forearm'] or ['Extensive damage to arteries or nerves? = true' and 'Fractured bone? = Wrist']] then*
'Perform surgery' has to be followed by 'Apply cast'

- *If[['Fractured bone? = Hand'] or ['Fractured bone? = Upper arm'] or ['Fractured bone? = Finger'] or ['Fractured bone? = Shoulder'] or ['Fractured bone? = Forearm'] or ['Fractured bone? = Wrist']] then*
'Apply sling' has to be performed at least 1 time

- *If[['In pain (now or in foreseeable future)? = true' and 'On anti-inflammatory drugs? = false' and 'On anticoagulants? = false' and 'On weak painkillers? = true']] then*
'Perform surgery' or 'Examine patient' have to be followed by 'Prescribe strong painkillers A'

- *If[['On anti-inflammatory drugs? = true' and 'In pain (now or in foreseeable future)? = true' and 'More than 16yrs old? = false' and 'On weak painkillers? = true'] or ['In pain (now or in foreseeable future)? = true' and 'More than 16yrs old? = true' and 'On anticoagulants? = true'] or ['On anti-inflammatory drugs? = true' and 'In pain (now or in foreseeable future)? = true' and 'More than 16yrs old? = true'] or ['In pain (now or in foreseeable future)? = true' and 'More than 16yrs old? = false' and 'On weak painkillers? = true' and 'On anticoagulants? = true']] then*
'Perform surgery' or 'Examine patient' have to be followed by 'Prescribe strong painkillers B'

- *If[['On weak painkillers? = false' and 'In pain (now or in foreseeable future)? = true' and 'More than 16yrs old? = false']] then*
'Perform surgery' or 'Examine patient' have to be followed by 'Prescribe weak painkillers'

- 'Perform surgery' has to be followed by 'Prescribe anticoagulants' within at most 4 h

- 'Perform surgery' has to be followed by 'Prescribe weak painkillers' or 'Prescribe strong painkillers B' within at most 4 h

- *If[['Fractured bone? = Shoulder' and 'Clear emergency? = false'] or ['Clear emergency? = false' and 'Fractured bone? = Hand'] or ['Clear emergency? = false' and 'Fractured bone? = Wrist'] or ['Clear emergency? = false' and 'Fractured bone? = Forearm'] or ['Clear emergency? = false' and 'Fractured bone? = Collarbone'] or ['Clear emergency? = false' and 'Fractured bone? = Finger'] or ['Clear emergency? = false' and 'Fractured bone? = Upper arm']] then*

'Take X-ray' has to precede 'Apply figure of eight bandage' or 'Apply fixation' or 'Apply cast' or 'Perform surgery'
- 'Apply cast' has to be followed by 'Perform surgery' or 'Take X-ray'
- *If[['Fractured bone? = Shoulder']] then*
  'Perform surgery' has to be followed by 'Perform physiotherapy'

Appendix C: Semi-structured Interview Protocol (Translated from Dutch)

Semi-structured interview:

A) Introduction
   1. Introduction of myself
   2. Description of the research project

      a. Knowledge-intensive, human-centric and flexible processes (like many processes in healthcare) are processes with a large set of activities that can be executed in many (infinite?) different sequences (= variations). For example...
      b. Doctors and nurses execute the process. They decide which activities to execute and when.
      c. To make decisions, they use what is called tacit knowledge: an implicit idea of how the process should be executed in each specific set of conditions.
      d. Implicit idea is based partially on explicit knowledge, but also for a large part on experience.
      e. Currently, no language supports all aspects of these processes to model them in sufficiently detail (= contain all important pieces of information and therefore convert implicit/tacit knowledge to explicit knowledge).
      f. Not being able to model them causes there to be a lack of transparency, but also little uniformity in the offered service (+lack of analysis).
      g. Made a language based on the identified needs.
      h. Now evaluating the result (= *language, not the actual model!*)
      i. Project with AZMM emergency department in the next phase

   3. Description of language

      a. General idea behind it

         i. Figures imperative vs declarative
         ii. Rules not enough, decisions are key (= context data)
             E.g., when do a blood test?

             1. Preventative to determine the general health status of a patient
             2. When suspecting a disease that shows in the bloodwork

         iii. Resources: available personnel, infrastructure and materials

      b. Going over the type of rules

         i. 4 big groups of templates
         ii. Examples...

4. Paint picture of scope of the case

    a. <u>Orthopedic</u> department: only diagnosis and treatment of patients with (suspected) fractures in their finger, hand, wrist, underarm, upper arm, shoulder and collarbone.

    b. Model originally created with nothing more than information available freely online

5. Introduction of the DeciClare textual model of the case

    a. Let them read the description
    b. Go over model elements
    c. Explain meaning of more complex rules

B) Evaluation of the model
  1. Semantic quality

    a. Is the model correct?
    b. Is the model complete?

       i. Amputation?
      ii. Medication?
     iii. Other tests (e.g., feel, test mobility…)?
     iv. Other treatments?
      v. Other decisions?

    c. Do the examples conform with the model?

       i. Yes
      ii. No:

        • Consult after X-ray
        • Rest after surgery
        • Cast after surgery

  2. Pragmatic quality

    a. Would the model be <u>useful</u> to support your daily tasks?
    b. Do you use <u>information like in the model</u> when making decisions?
    c. <u>How</u> do you use the described knowledge during the execution of the process? Is this similar to the type of rules in the model (implicit or explicit) or in some completely different manner?

C) Evaluation language
  1. Do you think that you could <u>learn</u> something from models like this?
  2. Do you think that the language is <u>sufficiently expressive</u> to model <u>similar</u> processes (e.g., the complete emergency medicine department)?

3. Do you know any rules or pieces of knowledge in this case or other healthcare processes that you think <u>cannot be modeled with the proposed language</u>?
4. Do you think that modeling these kinds of processes with such a language is <u>useful</u>? Could it be of <u>added value</u> to doctors and nurses, here and in general?

D) End

Appendix D: Final Textual DeciClare Model of Arm Fracture Case

The formal model is available at:
github.com/stevmert/DeciClareBPMS/blob/master/engine/models/ArmFractureCase_
DeciClareModel.txt

Defined Elements

- Available resources (13):
- [nurse(OR nurse), doctor(anesthesiologist/orthopedic surgeon/emergency doctor), receptionist, surgical assistant, reception desk, examination room, X-ray room, CT room, operating room, patient room, patient bed, recovery room, recovery bed]
- Available activities (25):
- [Register patient, Take medical history of patient, Clinical examination of patient, Doctor consultation, Take X-ray, Take CT scan, Prescribe NSAID painkillers, Prescribe SAID painkillers, Prescribe anticoagulants, Prescribe stomach protecting drug, Prescribe rest (= no treatment), Apply ice, Apply cast, Remove cast, Apply splint, Apply sling, Apply fixation, Remove fixation, Apply bandage, Apply figure of eight bandage, Perform surgery, Apply intra-compartmental pressure monitor, Let patient rest, Stay in patient room, Unregister patient]
- Available data records (2):
- [Patient File, Real-time observations]
- Available data attributes (21):
- [name = String, status = String, Patient has been to this hospital before? = (True/False), Is life-threatening emergency? = (True/False), Is conscious? = (True/False), Were there complications during surgery? = (True/False), Displaced fracture? = (True/False), Unstable fracture? = (True/False), Open fracture? = (True/False), More than 14yrs old? = (True/False), Bedridden patient? = (True/False), Operating time available? = (True/False), In pain? = (True/False), Is swollen? = (True/False), Numbness? = (True/False), Pin-and-needles? = (True/False), Has compartment syndrome? = (True/False), Has acute compartment syndrome? = (True/False), Needs surgery? = (True/False), Confirmed Fracture? = (Wrist/Forearm/Shoulder/Finger/Upper arm/Hand/Collarbone), Suspected fracture? = (Wrist/Forearm/Shoulder/Finger/Upper arm/Hand/Collarbone)]

Constraints

Data Constraints

- If[['Patient has been to this hospital before? = false']] then Register patient has to insert 'Patient File'
- If[['Patient has been to this hospital before? = false']] then Register patient has to insert 'Patient File -> name'

- If[['Patient has been to this hospital before? = false']] then Register patient has to insert 'Patient File -> status'
- If[['Patient has been to this hospital before? = true']] then Register patient has to read 'Patient File'
- If[['Patient has been to this hospital before? = false']] then Register patient has to read 'Patient File -> name'
- If[['Patient has been to this hospital before? = true']] then Register patient has to update 'Patient File -> status'
- Unregister patient has to update 'Patient File -> status'

Resource Constraints

- there is at least 1 receptionist available
- there are at most 2 receptionists available
- receptionist can be used by up to 1 instance(s) simultaneously
- OPTIONAL there are at least 4 nurses available
- there are at most 10 nurses available
- nurse(OR nurse) can be used by up to 1 instance(s) simultaneously
- OPTIONAL there is at least 1 OR nurse available
- doctor(anesthesiologist/orthopedic surgeon/emergency doctor) can be used by up to 1 instance(s) simultaneously
- OPTIONAL there is at least 1 emergency doctor available
- there are at most 5 emergency doctors available
- OPTIONAL there is at least 1 anesthesiologist available
- there are at most 2 anesthesiologists available
- OPTIONAL there is at least 1 orthopedic surgeon available
- there are at most 3 orthopedic surgeons available
- OPTIONAL there is at least 1 surgical assistant available
- there are at most 4 surgical assistants available
- surgical assistant can be used by up to 1 instance(s) simultaneously
- there is at least 1 reception desk available
- there are at most 2 reception desks available
- reception desk can be used by up to 1 instance(s) simultaneously
- OPTIONAL there are at least 3 examination rooms available
- there are at most 15 examination rooms available
- examination room can be used by up to 1 instance(s) simultaneously
- there is at least 1 operating room available
- there are at most 3 operating rooms available
- operating room can be used by up to 1 instance(s) simultaneously
- OPTIONAL there is at least 1 X-ray room available
- there are at most 2 X-ray rooms available
- X-ray room can be used by up to 1 instance(s) simultaneously
- there is at most 1 CT room available
- CT room can be used by up to 1 instance(s) simultaneously
- OPTIONAL there are at least 2 recovery beds available
- there are at most 10 recovery beds available
- recovery bed can be used by up to 1 instance(s) simultaneously

- there is at least 1 recovery room available
- there is at most 1 recovery room available
- recovery room can be used by up to 10 instance(s) simultaneously
- OPTIONAL there are at least 5 patient beds available
- there are at most 100 patient beds available
- patient bed can be used by up to 1 instance(s) simultaneously
- there are at most 50 patient rooms available
- patient room can be used by up to 2 instance(s) simultaneously
- a receptionist has authorization over Register patient
- Register patient uses at least 1 receptionist
- Register patient uses at most 1 receptionist
- Register patient uses at least 1 reception desk
- Register patient uses at most 1 reception desk
- a receptionist has authorization over Unregister patient
- Unregister patient uses at least 1 receptionist
- Unregister patient uses at most 1 receptionist
- Unregister patient uses at least 1 reception desk
- Unregister patient uses at most 1 reception desk
- a doctor or nurse have authorization over Take medical history of patient
- Take medical history of patient uses at least 1 doctor or nurse
- a doctor has authorization over Clinical examination of patient
- If[['Is life-threatening emergency? = false']] then Clinical examination of patient uses at least 1 examination room
- the decision of 'If[['Is life-threatening emergency? = false']] then Clinical examination of patient uses at least 1 examination room' has to be taken by a doctor
- Clinical examination of patient uses at least 1 doctor
- a doctor has authorization over Doctor consultation
- Doctor consultation uses at least 1 examination room
- Doctor consultation uses at least 1 doctor
- a doctor has authorization over Take X-ray
- Take X-ray uses at least 1 X-ray room
- Take X-ray uses at least 1 doctor or nurse
- OPTIONAL Take X-ray uses at least 1 nurse
- a doctor has authorization over Take CT scan
- Take CT scan uses at least 1 CT room
- Take CT scan uses at most 1 CT room
- Take CT scan uses at least 1 doctor or nurse
- OPTIONAL Take CT scan uses at least 1 nurse
- a doctor has authorization over Apply cast
- Apply cast uses at least 1 examination room
- Apply cast uses at most 1 examination room
- Apply cast uses at least 1 doctor or nurse
- OPTIONAL Apply cast uses at least 1 nurse
- a doctor has authorization over Remove cast
- Remove cast uses at least 1 examination room

- Remove cast uses at most 1 examination room
- Remove cast uses at least 1 doctor or nurse
- OPTIONAL Remove cast uses at least 1 nurse
- a doctor has authorization over Apply fixation
- Apply fixation uses at least 1 operating room
- Apply fixation uses at most 1 operating room
- Apply fixation uses at least 1 orthopedic surgeon
- Apply fixation uses at least 1 scrub nurse or surgical assistant
- Apply fixation uses at least 1 anesthesiologist
- Apply fixation uses at least 1 OR nurse
- OPTIONAL Apply fixation uses at least 2 OR nurse
- a doctor has authorization over Remove fixation
- Remove fixation uses at least 1 operating room
- Remove fixation uses at most 1 operating room
- Remove fixation uses at least 1 orthopedic surgeon
- Remove fixation uses at least 1 scrub nurse or surgical assistant
- Remove fixation uses at least 1 anesthesiologist
- Remove fixation uses at least 1 OR nurse
- OPTIONAL Remove fixation uses at least 2 OR nurse
- a doctor has authorization over Apply figure of eight bandage
- Apply figure of eight bandage uses at least 1 examination room
- Apply figure of eight bandage uses at most 1 examination room
- Apply figure of eight bandage uses at least 1 doctor or nurse
- OPTIONAL Apply figure of eight bandage uses at least 1 nurse
- a doctor or nurse have authorization over Apply bandage
- Apply bandage uses at least 1 doctor or nurse
- OPTIONAL Apply bandage uses at least 1 nurse
- a doctor or nurse have authorization over Apply splint
- Apply splint uses at least 1 doctor or nurse
- OPTIONAL Apply splint uses at least 1 nurse
- a doctor or nurse have authorization over Apply sling
- Apply sling uses at least 1 doctor or nurse
- OPTIONAL Apply sling uses at least 1 nurse
- a doctor or nurse have authorization over Apply ice
- a doctor has authorization over Perform surgery
- Perform surgery uses at least 1 operating room
- Perform surgery uses at most 1 operating room
- Perform surgery uses at least 1 orthopedic surgeon
- Perform surgery uses at least 1 scrub nurse or surgical assistant
- Perform surgery uses at least 1 anesthesiologist
- Perform surgery uses at least 1 OR nurse
- OPTIONAL Perform surgery uses at least 2 OR nurse
- a doctor has authorization over Apply intra-compartmental pressure monitor
- Apply intra-compartmental pressure monitor uses at least 1 doctor or nurse
- a doctor has authorization over Let patient rest
- Let patient rest uses at least 1 recovery bed

- Let patient rest uses at most 1 recovery bed
- Let patient rest uses at least 1 recovery room
- Let patient rest uses at most 1 recovery room
- Stay in patient room uses at least 1 patient bed
- Stay in patient room uses at most 1 patient bed
- Stay in patient room uses at least 1 patient room
- Stay in patient room uses at most 1 patient room
- a doctor has authorization over Prescribe NSAID painkillers
- a doctor has authorization over Prescribe SAID painkillers
- a doctor has authorization over Prescribe anticoagulants
- a doctor has authorization over Prescribe stomach protecting drug
- a doctor has authorization over Prescribe rest (= no treatment)
- the following resources cannot be equal: orthopedic surgeon in Apply fixation or Perform surgery or Remove fixation, anesthesiologist in Apply fixation or Perform surgery or Remove fixation

Functional/Control-flow Constraints

- If[['Is life-threatening emergency? = false']] then (Register patient has to be performed at least 1 time) has to precede (Take medical history of patient has to be performed at least 1 time)
- If[['Is life-threatening emergency? = false']] then (Register patient has to be performed at least 1 time) has to precede (Clinical examination of patient has to be performed at least 1 time)
- If[['Is life-threatening emergency? = false']] then (Register patient has to be performed at least 1 time) has to precede (Doctor consultation has to be performed at least 1 time)
- If[['Is life-threatening emergency? = false']] then (Register patient has to be performed at least 1 time) has to precede (Take X-ray has to be performed at least 1 time)
- If[['Is life-threatening emergency? = false']] then (Register patient has to be performed at least 1 time) has to precede (Take CT scan has to be performed at least 1 time)
- If[['Is life-threatening emergency? = false']] then (Register patient has to be performed at least 1 time) has to precede (Prescribe NSAID painkillers has to be performed at least 1 time)
- If[['Is life-threatening emergency? = false']] then (Register patient has to be performed at least 1 time) has to precede (Prescribe SAID painkillers has to be performed at least 1 time)
- If[['Is life-threatening emergency? = false']] then (Register patient has to be performed at least 1 time) has to precede (Prescribe anticoagulants has to be performed at least 1 time)
- If[['Is life-threatening emergency? = false']] then (Register patient has to be performed at least 1 time) has to precede (Prescribe stomach protecting drug has to be performed at least 1 time)

- If[['Is life-threatening emergency? = false']] then (Register patient has to be performed at least 1 time) has to precede (Prescribe rest (= no treatment) has to be performed at least 1 time)
- If[['Is life-threatening emergency? = false']] then (Register patient has to be performed at least 1 time) has to precede (Apply ice has to be performed at least 1 time)
- If[['Is life-threatening emergency? = false']] then (Register patient has to be performed at least 1 time) has to precede (Apply cast has to be performed at least 1 time)
- If[['Is life-threatening emergency? = false']] then (Register patient has to be performed at least 1 time) has to precede (Remove cast has to be performed at least 1 time)
- If[['Is life-threatening emergency? = false']] then (Register patient has to be performed at least 1 time) has to precede (Apply splint has to be performed at least 1 time)
- If[['Is life-threatening emergency? = false']] then (Register patient has to be performed at least 1 time) has to precede (Apply sling has to be performed at least 1 time)
- If[['Is life-threatening emergency? = false']] then (Register patient has to be performed at least 1 time) has to precede (Apply fixation has to be performed at least 1 time)
- If[['Is life-threatening emergency? = false']] then (Register patient has to be performed at least 1 time) has to precede (Remove fixation has to be performed at least 1 time)
- If[['Is life-threatening emergency? = false']] then (Register patient has to be performed at least 1 time) has to precede (Apply bandage has to be performed at least 1 time)
- If[['Is life-threatening emergency? = false']] then (Register patient has to be performed at least 1 time) has to precede (Apply figure of eight bandage has to be performed at least 1 time)
- If[['Is life-threatening emergency? = false']] then (Register patient has to be performed at least 1 time) has to precede (Perform surgery has to be performed at least 1 time)
- If[['Is life-threatening emergency? = false']] then (Register patient has to be performed at least 1 time) has to precede (Apply intra-compartmental pressure monitor has to be performed at least 1 time)
- If[['Is life-threatening emergency? = false']] then (Register patient has to be performed at least 1 time) has to precede (Let patient rest has to be performed at least 1 time)
- If[['Is life-threatening emergency? = false']] then (Register patient has to be performed at least 1 time) has to precede (Stay in patient room has to be performed at least 1 time)
- If[['Is life-threatening emergency? = false']] then (Register patient has to be performed at least 1 time) has to precede (Unregister patient has to be performed at least 1 time)

- (Register patient has to be performed at least 1 time) has to be followed by (Unregister patient has to be performed at least 1 time)
- (Take medical history of patient has to be performed at least 1 time) has to be followed by (Unregister patient has to be performed at least 1 time)
- (Clinical examination of patient has to be performed at least 1 time) has to be followed by (Unregister patient has to be performed at least 1 time)
- (Doctor consultation has to be performed at least 1 time) has to be followed by (Unregister patient has to be performed at least 1 time)
- (Take X-ray has to be performed at least 1 time) has to be followed by (Unregister patient has to be performed at least 1 time)
- (Take CT scan has to be performed at least 1 time) has to be followed by (Unregister patient has to be performed at least 1 time)
- (Prescribe NSAID painkillers has to be performed at least 1 time) has to be followed by (Unregister patient has to be performed at least 1 time)
- (Prescribe SAID painkillers has to be performed at least 1 time) has to be followed by (Unregister patient has to be performed at least 1 time)
- (Prescribe anticoagulants has to be performed at least 1 time) has to be followed by (Unregister patient has to be performed at least 1 time)
- (Prescribe stomach protecting drug has to be performed at least 1 time) has to be followed by (Unregister patient has to be performed at least 1 time)
- (Prescribe rest (= no treatment) has to be performed at least 1 time) has to be followed by (Unregister patient has to be performed at least 1 time)
- (Apply ice has to be performed at least 1 time) has to be followed by (Unregister patient has to be performed at least 1 time)
- (Apply cast has to be performed at least 1 time) has to be followed by (Unregister patient has to be performed at least 1 time)
- (Remove cast has to be performed at least 1 time) has to be followed by (Unregister patient has to be performed at least 1 time)
- (Apply splint has to be performed at least 1 time) has to be followed by (Unregister patient has to be performed at least 1 time)
- (Apply sling has to be performed at least 1 time) has to be followed by (Unregister patient has to be performed at least 1 time)
- (Apply fixation has to be performed at least 1 time) has to be followed by (Unregister patient has to be performed at least 1 time)
- (Remove fixation has to be performed at least 1 time) has to be followed by (Unregister patient has to be performed at least 1 time)
- (Apply bandage has to be performed at least 1 time) has to be followed by (Unregister patient has to be performed at least 1 time)
- (Apply figure of eight bandage has to be performed at least 1 time) has to be followed by (Unregister patient has to be performed at least 1 time)
- (Perform surgery has to be performed at least 1 time) has to be followed by (Unregister patient has to be performed at least 1 time)
- (Apply intra-compartmental pressure monitor has to be performed at least 1 time) has to be followed by (Unregister patient has to be performed at least 1 time)

- (Let patient rest has to be performed at least 1 time) has to be followed by (Unregister patient has to be performed at least 1 time)
- (Stay in patient room has to be performed at least 1 time) has to be followed by (Unregister patient has to be performed at least 1 time)
- Register patient has to be performed at least 1 time
- Register patient can be performed at most 1 time
- Unregister patient has to be performed at least 1 time
- Unregister patient can be performed at most 1 time
- (Clinical examination of patient has to be performed at least 1 time) has to precede (Stay in patient room has to be performed at least 1 time)
- If[['Is conscious? = true']] then Take medical history of patient has to be performed at least 1 time
- the decision of 'If[['Is conscious? = true']] then Take medical history of patient has to be performed at least 1 time' has to be taken by a doctor or nurse
- Clinical examination of patient has to be performed at least 1 time
- If[['Is conscious? = true']] then (Take medical history of patient has to be performed at least 1 time) has to precede (Clinical examination of patient has to be performed at least 1 time)
- the decision of 'If[['Is conscious? = true']] then (Take medical history of patient has to be performed at least 1 time) has to precede (Clinical examination of patient has to be performed at least 1 time)' has to be taken by a doctor or nurse
- If[['Is life-threatening emergency? = false']] then Take X-ray has to be performed at least 1 time
- the decision of 'If[['Is life-threatening emergency? = false']] then Take X-ray has to be performed at least 1 time' has to be taken by a doctor
- If[['Suspected fracture? = Shoulder'] or ['Confirmed Fracture? = Shoulder' and 'Needs surgery? = false']] then Take CT scan has to be performed at least 1 time
- the decision of 'If[['Suspected fracture? = Shoulder'] or ['Confirmed Fracture? = Shoulder' and 'Needs surgery? = false']] then Take CT scan has to be performed at least 1 time' has to be taken by a doctor
- Take CT scan is only available [Every Monday, between 8am and 6 pm]/[Every Tuesday, between 8am and 6 pm]/[Every Wednesday, between 8am and 5 pm]/ [Every Thursday, between 8am and 6 pm]/[Every Friday, between 8am and 6 pm]
- If[['In pain? = true' and 'Is swollen? = true' and 'Pin-and-needles? = true' and 'Suspected fracture? = Hand'] or ['In pain? = true' and 'Suspected fracture? = Forearm' and 'Is swollen? = true' and 'Pin-and-needles? = true'] or ['In pain? = true' and 'Is swollen? = true' and 'Pin-and-needles? = true' and 'Suspected fracture? = Upper arm']] then Apply intra-compartmental pressure monitor has to be performed at least 1 time within at most 30 min
- the decision of 'If[['In pain? = true' and 'Is swollen? = true' and 'Pin-and-needles? = true' and 'Suspected fracture? = Hand'] or ['In pain? = true' and 'Suspected fracture? = Forearm' and 'Is swollen? = true' and 'Pin-and-needles? = true'] or ['In pain? = true' and 'Is swollen? = true' and 'Pin-and-needles? = true' and 'Suspected fracture? = Upper arm']] then Apply

intra-compartmental pressure monitor has to be performed at least 1 time within at most 30 min' has to be taken by a doctor

- (Clinical examination of patient has to be performed at least 1 time) has to precede (Doctor consultation has to be performed at least 1 time)
- (Clinical examination of patient has to be performed at least 1 time) has to precede (Take X-ray has to be performed at least 1 time)
- (Clinical examination of patient has to be performed at least 1 time) has to precede (Take CT scan has to be performed at least 1 time)
- (Clinical examination of patient has to be performed at least 1 time) has to precede (Apply intra-compartmental pressure monitor has to be performed at least 1 time)
- (Take CT scan has to be performed at least 1 time) or (Take X-ray has to be performed at least 1 time) have to be followed by (Doctor consultation has to be performed at least 1 time)
- at least 1 out of 11 of the following activities have to be performed: Prescribe SAID painkillers or Prescribe rest (= no treatment) or Apply sling or Apply figure of eight bandage or Apply fixation or Apply ice or Prescribe NSAID painkillers or Perform surgery or Apply splint or Apply cast or Apply bandage
- (Clinical examination of patient has to be performed at least 1 time) has to precede (Prescribe NSAID painkillers has to be performed at least 1 time)
- (Clinical examination of patient has to be performed at least 1 time) has to precede (Prescribe SAID painkillers has to be performed at least 1 time)
- (Clinical examination of patient has to be performed at least 1 time) has to precede (Prescribe anticoagulants has to be performed at least 1 time)
- (Clinical examination of patient has to be performed at least 1 time) has to precede (Prescribe stomach protecting drug has to be performed at least 1 time)
- (Clinical examination of patient has to be performed at least 1 time) has to precede (Prescribe rest (= no treatment) has to be performed at least 1 time)
- (Clinical examination of patient has to be performed at least 1 time) has to precede (Apply cast has to be performed at least 1 time)
- (Clinical examination of patient has to be performed at least 1 time) has to precede (Apply fixation has to be performed at least 1 time)
- (Clinical examination of patient has to be performed at least 1 time) has to precede (Apply figure of eight bandage has to be performed at least 1 time)
- (Clinical examination of patient has to be performed at least 1 time) has to precede (Perform surgery has to be performed at least 1 time)
- OPTIONAL If[['Is swollen? = true'] or ['Has compartment syndrome? = true']] then Apply ice has to be performed at least 1 time unless If[['Is swollen? = false' and 'Has compartment syndrome? = false']]
- the decision of 'OPTIONAL If[['Is swollen? = true'] or ['Has compartment syndrome? = true']] then Apply ice has to be performed at least 1 time unless If [['Is swollen? = false' and 'Has compartment syndrome? = false']]' has to be taken by a doctor

- OPTIONAL before (Prescribe anticoagulants has to be performed at least 1 time) can be executed after the execution of (Prescribe NSAID painkillers has to be performed at least 1 time) at least 12 h have to have elapsed
- OPTIONAL before (Prescribe NSAID painkillers has to be performed at least 1 time) can be executed after the execution of (Prescribe anticoagulants has to be performed at least 1 time) at least 12 h have to have elapsed
- OPTIONAL (Prescribe anticoagulants has to be performed at least 1 time) has to be directly followed by (Prescribe stomach protecting drug has to be performed at least 1 time)
- OPTIONAL If[['In pain? = true']] then Prescribe SAID painkillers or Prescribe NSAID painkillers have to be performed at least a combined 1 time
- the decision of 'OPTIONAL If[['In pain? = true']] then Prescribe SAID painkillers or Prescribe NSAID painkillers have to be performed at least a combined 1 time' has to be taken by a doctor
- (Apply cast has to be performed at least 1 time) has to be followed by (Remove cast has to be performed at least 1 time)
- (Apply cast has to be performed at least 1 time) has to precede (Remove cast has to be performed at least 1 time)
- (Apply fixation has to be performed at least 1 time) has to be followed by (Remove fixation has to be performed at least 1 time)
- (Apply fixation has to be performed at least 1 time) has to precede (Remove fixation has to be performed at least 1 time)
- If[['Has compartment syndrome? = true']] then (Apply cast has to be performed at least 1 time) and (Remove cast can be performed at most 0 times) have to be followed by (Remove cast has to be performed at least 1 time) within at most 15 min
- the decision of 'If[['Has compartment syndrome? = true']] then (Apply cast has to be performed at least 1 time) and (Remove cast can be performed at most 0 times) have to be followed by (Remove cast has to be performed at least 1 time) within at most 15 min' has to be taken by a doctor
- If[['Has compartment syndrome? = true']] then (Apply fixation has to be performed at least 1 time) and (Remove fixation can be performed at most 0 times) have to be followed by (Remove fixation has to be performed at least 1 time) within at most 15 min
- the decision of 'If[['Has compartment syndrome? = true']] then (Apply fixation has to be performed at least 1 time) and (Remove fixation can be performed at most 0 times) have to be followed by (Remove fixation has to be performed at least 1 time) within at most 15 min' has to be taken by a doctor
- If[['Displaced fracture? = true' and 'Operating time available? = false' and 'Confirmed Fracture? = Wrist'] or ['Displaced fracture? = true' and 'Operating time available? = false' and 'Confirmed Fracture? = Forearm']] then ((Apply cast has to be performed at least 1 time) or (Apply splint has to be performed at least 1 time)) and (Stay in patient room has to be performed at least 1 time) have to precede (Perform surgery has to be performed at least 1 time) unless If [['Operating time available? = true']]

- the decision of 'If[['Displaced fracture? = true' and 'Operating time available? = false' and 'Confirmed Fracture? = Wrist'] or ['Displaced fracture? = true' and 'Operating time available? = false' and 'Confirmed Fracture? = Forearm']] then ((Apply cast has to be performed at least 1 time) or (Apply splint has to be performed at least 1 time)) and (Stay in patient room has to be performed at least 1 time) have to precede (Perform surgery has to be performed at least 1 time) unless If[['Operating time available? = true']]' has to be taken by a doctor
- If[['Confirmed Fracture? = Shoulder'] or ['Confirmed Fracture? = Upper arm'] or ['Confirmed Fracture? = Forearm'] or ['Confirmed Fracture? = Wrist'] or ['Confirmed Fracture? = Finger'] or ['Confirmed Fracture? = Hand']] then Apply sling has to be performed at least 1 time
- the decision of 'If[['Confirmed Fracture? = Shoulder'] or ['Confirmed Fracture? = Upper arm'] or ['Confirmed Fracture? = Forearm'] or ['Confirmed Fracture? = Wrist'] or ['Confirmed Fracture? = Finger'] or ['Confirmed Fracture? = Hand']] then Apply sling has to be performed at least 1 time' has to be taken by a doctor or nurse
- If[['Open fracture? = false' and 'Confirmed Fracture? = Forearm' and 'Displaced fracture? = false'] or ['Confirmed Fracture? = Shoulder' and 'Open fracture? = false' and 'Displaced fracture? = false'] or ['Open fracture? = false' and 'More than 14yrs old? = true' and 'Displaced fracture? = false' and 'Confirmed Fracture? = Wrist']] then Apply cast or Apply splint have to be performed at least a combined 1 time
- the decision of 'If[['Open fracture? = false' and 'Confirmed Fracture? = Forearm' and 'Displaced fracture? = false'] or ['Confirmed Fracture? = Shoulder' and 'Open fracture? = false' and 'Displaced fracture? = false'] or ['Open fracture? = false' and 'More than 14yrs old? = true' and 'Displaced fracture? = false' and 'Confirmed Fracture? = Wrist']] then Apply cast or Apply splint have to be performed at least a combined 1 time' has to be taken by a doctor
- If[['Confirmed Fracture? = Finger' and 'Unstable fracture? = false' and 'Open fracture? = false' and 'Displaced fracture? = false']] then Apply splint and Apply bandage have to be performed at least a combined 1 time
- the decision of 'If[['Confirmed Fracture? = Finger' and 'Unstable fracture? = false' and 'Open fracture? = false' and 'Displaced fracture? = false']] then Apply splint and Apply bandage have to be performed at least a combined 1 time' has to be taken by a doctor
- If[['Confirmed Fracture? = Finger' and 'Open fracture? = true'] or ['Confirmed Fracture? = Finger' and 'Displaced fracture? = true'] or ['Confirmed Fracture? = Finger' and 'Unstable fracture? = true']] then Apply fixation has to be performed at least 1 time
- the decision of 'If[['Confirmed Fracture? = Finger' and 'Open fracture? = true'] or ['Confirmed Fracture? = Finger' and 'Displaced fracture? = true'] or ['Confirmed Fracture? = Finger' and 'Unstable fracture? = true']] then Apply fixation has to be performed at least 1 time' has to be taken by a doctor

- If[['Unstable fracture? = false' and 'Open fracture? = false' and 'Displaced fracture? = false' and 'Confirmed Fracture? = Hand']] then Apply fixation or Apply splint or Apply cast have to be performed at least a combined 1 time
- the decision of 'If[['Unstable fracture? = false' and 'Open fracture? = false' and 'Displaced fracture? = false' and 'Confirmed Fracture? = Hand']] then Apply fixation or Apply splint or Apply cast have to be performed at least a combined 1 time' has to be taken by a doctor
- If[['Unstable fracture? = false' and 'Confirmed Fracture? = Upper arm' and 'Open fracture? = false' and 'Displaced fracture? = false']] then Apply sling or Apply cast or Apply splint have to be performed at least a combined 1 time
- the decision of 'If[['Unstable fracture? = false' and 'Confirmed Fracture? = Upper arm' and 'Open fracture? = false' and 'Displaced fracture? = false']] then Apply sling or Apply cast or Apply splint have to be performed at least a combined 1 time' has to be taken by a doctor
- If[['Unstable fracture? = false' and 'Open fracture? = false' and 'Displaced fracture? = false' and 'Confirmed Fracture? = Collarbone']] then Apply figure of eight bandage or Apply splint have to be performed at least a combined 1 time
- the decision of 'If[['Unstable fracture? = false' and 'Open fracture? = false' and 'Displaced fracture? = false' and 'Confirmed Fracture? = Collarbone']] then Apply figure of eight bandage or Apply splint have to be performed at least a combined 1 time' has to be taken by a doctor
- OPTIONAL If[['Confirmed Fracture? = Collarbone']] then Apply sling has to be performed at least 1 time
- the decision of 'OPTIONAL If[['Confirmed Fracture? = Collarbone']] then Apply sling has to be performed at least 1 time' has to be taken by a doctor or nurse
- If[['Is life-threatening emergency? = false' and 'Suspected fracture? = Shoulder']] then Take X-ray or Take CT scan have to be performed at least a combined 1 time
- the decision of 'If[['Is life-threatening emergency? = false' and 'Suspected fracture? = Shoulder']] then Take X-ray or Take CT scan have to be performed at least a combined 1 time' has to be taken by a doctor
- If[['Confirmed Fracture? = Shoulder']] then Take X-ray has to be performed at least 1 time after at least 1 day
- the decision of 'If[['Confirmed Fracture? = Shoulder']] then Take X-ray has to be performed at least 1 time after at least 1 day' has to be taken by a doctor
- OPTIONAL If[['Confirmed Fracture? = Shoulder' and 'Open fracture? = false' and 'Displaced fracture? = false']] then Perform surgery can be performed at most 0 times
- the decision of 'OPTIONAL If[['Confirmed Fracture? = Shoulder' and 'Open fracture? = false' and 'Displaced fracture? = false']] then Perform surgery can be performed at most 0 times' has to be taken by a doctor
- If[['Were there complications during surgery? = false']] then (Perform surgery has to be performed at least 1 time) has to be followed by (Let patient rest has to be performed at least 1 time) within at most 5 min

- the decision of 'If[['Were there complications during surgery? = false']] then (Perform surgery has to be performed at least 1 time) has to be followed by (Let patient rest has to be performed at least 1 time) within at most 5 min' has to be taken by a doctor
- If[['Displaced fracture? = true'] or ['Open fracture? = true']] then Perform surgery has to be performed at least 1 time
- the decision of 'If[['Displaced fracture? = true'] or ['Open fracture? = true']] then Perform surgery has to be performed at least 1 time' has to be taken by a doctor
- If[['Has acute compartment syndrome? = true']] then Perform surgery has to be performed at least 1 time within at most 1 h
- the decision of 'If[['Has acute compartment syndrome? = true']] then Perform surgery has to be performed at least 1 time within at most 1 h' has to be taken by a doctor
- If[['Unstable fracture? = true']] then Perform surgery or (Take X-ray and Doctor consultation) have to be performed at least a combined 1 time
- the decision of 'If[['Unstable fracture? = true']] then Perform surgery or (Take X-ray and Doctor consultation) have to be performed at least a combined 1 time' has to be taken by a doctor
- (Perform surgery has to be performed at least 1 time) has to be followed by (Prescribe NSAID painkillers has to be performed at least 1 time) or ((Prescribe SAID painkillers has to be performed at least 1 time) and (Prescribe anticoagulants has to be performed at least 1 time)) within at most 4 h
- If[['Bedridden patient? = true']] then (Perform surgery has to be performed at least 1 time) has to be followed by (Prescribe SAID painkillers has to be performed at least 1 time) and (Prescribe anticoagulants has to be performed at least 1 time) within at most 4 h
- the decision of 'If[['Bedridden patient? = true']] then (Perform surgery has to be performed at least 1 time) has to be followed by (Prescribe SAID painkillers has to be performed at least 1 time) and (Prescribe anticoagulants has to be performed at least 1 time) within at most 4 h' has to be taken by a doctor
- (Apply cast has to be performed at least 1 time) has to be followed by (Perform surgery has to be performed at least 1 time) or (Take X-ray has to be performed at least 1 time)
- If[['Open fracture? = true' and 'Confirmed Fracture? = Forearm'] or ['Open fracture? = true' and 'Confirmed Fracture? = Wrist'] or ['Displaced fracture? = true' and 'Confirmed Fracture? = Wrist'] or ['Displaced fracture? = true' and 'Confirmed Fracture? = Forearm']] then (Perform surgery has to be performed at least 1 time) has to be followed by (Apply cast has to be performed at least 1 time) or (Apply splint has to be performed at least 1 time)
- the decision of 'If[['Open fracture? = true' and 'Confirmed Fracture? = Forearm'] or ['Open fracture? = true' and 'Confirmed Fracture? = Wrist'] or ['Displaced fracture? = true' and 'Confirmed Fracture? = Wrist'] or ['Displaced fracture? = true' and 'Confirmed Fracture? = Forearm']] then (Perform surgery has to be performed at least 1

time) has to be followed by (Apply cast has to be performed at least 1 time) or (Apply splint has to be performed at least 1 time)' has to be taken by a doctor

- If[['Is life-threatening emergency? = false' and 'Suspected fracture? = Hand'] or ['Suspected fracture? = Finger' and 'Is life-threatening emergency? = false'] or ['Is life-threatening emergency? = false' and 'Suspected fracture? = Upper arm'] or ['Is life-threatening emergency? = false' and 'Suspected fracture? = Collarbone'] or ['Is life-threatening emergency? = false' and 'Suspected fracture? = Forearm'] or ['Is life-threatening emergency? = false' and 'Suspected fracture? = Wrist']] then (Take X-ray has to be performed at least 1 time) has to precede (Apply fixation has to be performed at least 1 time) or (Apply cast has to be performed at least 1 time) or (Apply figure of eight bandage has to be performed at least 1 time) or (Perform surgery has to be performed at least 1 time)

- the decision of 'If[['Is life-threatening emergency? = false' and 'Suspected fracture? = Hand'] or ['Suspected fracture? = Finger' and 'Is life-threatening emergency? = false'] or ['Is life-threatening emergency? = false' and 'Suspected fracture? = Upper arm'] or ['Is life-threatening emergency? = false' and 'Suspected fracture? = Collarbone'] or ['Is life-threatening emergency? = false' and 'Suspected fracture? = Forearm'] or ['Is life-threatening emergency? = false' and 'Suspected fracture? = Wrist']] then (Take X-ray has to be performed at least 1 time) has to precede (Apply fixation has to be performed at least 1 time) or (Apply cast has to be performed at least 1 time) or (Apply figure of eight bandage has to be performed at least 1 time) or (Perform surgery has to be performed at least 1 time)' has to be taken by a doctor

- OPTIONAL If[['In pain? = true']] then (Prescribe anticoagulants can be performed at most 0 times) and ((Doctor consultation has to be performed at least 1 time) or (Clinical examination of patient has to be performed at least 1 time) or (Perform surgery has to be performed at least 1 time)) have to be directly followed by (Prescribe NSAID painkillers has to be performed at least 1 time)

- the decision of 'OPTIONAL If[['In pain? = true']] then (Prescribe anticoagulants can be performed at most 0 times) and ((Doctor consultation has to be performed at least 1 time) or (Clinical examination of patient has to be performed at least 1 time) or (Perform surgery has to be performed at least 1 time)) have to be directly followed by (Prescribe NSAID painkillers has to be performed at least 1 time)' has to be taken by a doctor

Appendix E: The Join Step of DeciClareMiner (Decision-Independent)

Rules with a logical expression of size k are joined to create rules with a logical expression of size k + 1 in the iteration steps of the algorithm. However, the elements of the logical expressions can be connected with either the inclusive disjunction or the logical conjunction operator. Therefore, the influence of joining these logical expressions using either operator on the number of violations and the support level has been investigated for each template to apply the leveraged property.

The relation constraint templates have two possible logical expressions that can be joined: joining the logical expressions on the condition sides of relation constraints and joining the logical expressions on the consequence sides. Table A.1 and Table A.2 present the lower and upper bound for the number of conforming (#C) and violating (#V) occurrences of the child rule relative to the respective values for the parent rules for each type of join operation. For example, consider rules Response(AtLeast(A, 1), AtLeast(B, 1)) and Response(AtLeast(A, 1), AtLeast(C, 1)) for an event log consisting of four times trace 'AB' and two times 'AC'. The former rule has 4 confirming and 2 violating occurrences, while the latter has 2 confirming and 4 violating occurrences. Table A.2 states that the rule resulting from the OR-join operation on the consequence side, Response(AtLeast(A, 1), AtLeast(B or C, 1)), will have at least 4 (= max[4, 2]) and at most 6 (= min[4 + 2, 6]) confirming occurrences and at least 0 (= max[6-6, 0]) and at most 2 (= min[4, 2]) violating occurrences. Evaluating the rule results in 6 confirming occurrences and no violations.

A distinction is also made between the positive (i.e., 'at least …' consequence) and negative (i.e., 'at most 0' consequence) versions of the relation templates, as this allows for more specific bounds.

Based on Table A.1 and Table A.2, optimizations can be formulated for the join operations for each type of relation rule. At the condition side, it is clear that the OR-join will never result in a minimal rule as the number of violations of the child rule is at least equal to the highest number of violations of its parent rules. So only the

Table A.1. The bounds for join operation of the condition side of the relation templates.

	'At least 1' consequence expression		'At most 0' consequence expression	
	OR-join	AND-join	OR-join	AND-join
Max #C	sum(#C)	min(#C)	sum(#C)	min(#C)
Min #C	max(#C)	0	max(#C)	0
Max #V	sum(#V)	min(#V)	sum(#V)	min(#V)
Min #V	max(#V)	0	max(#V)	0

Table A.2. The bounds for join operation of the consequence side of the relation templates.

	'At least 1' consequence expression		'At most 0' consequence expression	
	OR-join	AND-join	OR-join	AND-join
Max #C	min(sum(#C), #Occurrences)	min(#C)	min(#C)	min(sum(#C), #Occurrences)
Min #C	max(#C)	max(sum(#C) - #Occurrences, 0)	max(sum(#C) - #Occurrences, 0)	max(#C)
Max #V	min(#V)	min(sum(#V), #Occurrences)	min(sum(#V), #Occurrences)	min(#V)
Min #V	max(sum(#V) - #Occurrences, 0)	max(#V)	max(#V)	max(sum(#V) - #Occurrences, 0)

AND-join operation will be used when joining condition sides. Additionally, these bounds make it possible to know beforehand if the resulting rule can have a support level higher than the threshold. The maximum support level of the child rule is the sum of the maximal number of conforming occurrences and the maximal number of violating occurrences. In this case, this is equal to the sum of the minimal number of conforming occurrences and the minimal number of violating occurrences of the parent rules. A similar conclusion can be drawn at the consequence side, however, the join operation to use now depends on whether or not the constraint in question is based on a positive or a negative relation template. Positive constraints will only use the OR-join, while negative constraints will only use the AND-join. The bounds for the consequence side do not allow for any conclusions to be drawn about the support level of the child rule.

Additionally, the iteration step will be executed twice for relation templates, because the join operations are defined for the condition and consequence side separately. The first time it will be executed with the input described in the initialization step. This will only grow the size of the condition side logical expression of the constraints. The resulting output is a set of all the minimal rules that occur at least once with a consequence side logical expression of length one. This output is then again used as input for the algorithm, but this time the consequence side logical expression is the one that is allowed to grow.

The proposed algorithm only supports two of the resource templates, namely the AtLeastUsage1 and AtMostUsage0 templates, as the others are difficult to mine from traditional event logs. For these two templates, the bounds for the number of confirming and violating occurrences of this join operation are the same as for the positive relation templates in Table A.1.

Appendix F: The DeciClare Templates Supported by DeciClareEngine

The current implementation of the DeciClareEngine-tool supports the 18 most important constraint templates of DeciClare. Support for more templates will be added later. Table A.3 presents the currently supported constraint templates, each of which is accompanied by an example that illustrates its meaning and parameters. The parameters I and B define the logical operators that can be used in the parameter expressions of the template because of branching. The letter used refers to the option of using either the inclusive disjunction (I) or both the inclusive disjunction and conjunction (B).

Although supported by the DeciClareEngine, Table A.3 omits the timing parameters required for each of the templates, except for the untimed RespondedPresence, AtLeastLag and ActivityAuthorization templates, to avoid overloading the table. These are two parameters expressing the time interval in which the constraint applies. For example, Response(AtLeast(e1, 1), AtLeast(e2, 1), 2, 7) expresses that if e1 is executed, then e2 must be executed at least once after at least 2 time units and at most 7 time units after e1 was executed. The lower- and upper-bound time parameters can be 0 and infinity, respectively, reducing them to the examples presented in Table A.3.

Similarly, activation decisions are omitted in Table A.3 but supported by DeciClareEngine. The deactivation decisions are not yet supported.

Table A.3. The constraint templates supported by DeciClareEngine.

Class	Template	Example
Existence	AtLeast(I, n)	AtLeast(Apply bandage or Apply cast, 2): the sum of the occurrences of Apply bandage and the occurrences of Apply cast has to be at least 2
	AtMost(B, n)	AtMost(Examine patient and Take X-ray, 3): the number of co-occurrences of Examine patient and Take X-ray must be at most 3
	AtLeastChoice(B, n)	AtLeastChoice(Prescribe SAID painkillers or Prescribe NSAID painkillers, 1): at least one of the two activities has to be executed (independent of how many times)
	AtMostChoice(B, n)	AtMostChoice(Prescribe SAID painkillers or Prescribe anticoagulants, 1): at most one of the two activities can to be executed (independent of how many times)
	First(I)	First(Register patient, Examine patient): either Register patient or Examine patient has to be executed before any other event can be executed
	Last(I)	Last(Apply sling or Examine patient): either Apply sling or Examine patient has to be executed as the final event
Relation	RespondedPresence(B_1, B_2)	RespondedPresence(AtLeast((Take X-ray and Apply sling) or Apply bandage, 1), AtLeast(Examine patient

(continued)

Table A.3. (*Continued*)

Class	Template	Example
		or Perform surgery, 1)): if Take X-ray and Apply sling or just Apply bandage are executed at least once, then Examine patient or Perform surgery must also be executed at least once somewhere in the instance (before, during or after)
	Response(B_1, B_2)	Response(AtLeast((Take X-ray and Apply sling) or Apply bandage, 1), AtLeast(Examine patient or Perform surgery, 1)): if Take X-ray and Apply sling or just Apply bandage are executed at least once, then Examine patient or Perform surgery must also be executed at least once at some time after Take X-ray and Apply sling or after Apply bandage
	ChainResponse(B_1, B_2)	ChainResponse(AtLeast((Take X-ray and Apply sling) or Apply bandage, 1), AtLeast(Examine patient or Perform surgery, 1)): if Take X-ray and Apply sling or just Apply bandage are/is executed at least once, then Examine patient or Perform surgery must also be executed at least once immediately after Take X-ray and Apply sling or after Apply bandage
	Precedence(B_1, B_2)	Precedence(AtLeast((Take X-ray and Apply sling) or Apply bandage, 1), AtLeast(Examine patient or Perform surgery, 1)): Take X-ray and Apply sling or just Apply bandage can be executed only after Examine patient or Perform surgery has already been executed at least once
	ChainPrecedence(B_1, B_2)	ChainPrecedence(AtLeast((Take X-ray and Apply sling) or Apply bandage, 1), AtLeast(Examine patient or Perform surgery, 1)): Take X-ray and Apply sling or just Apply bandage can be executed only immediately after Examine patient or Perform surgery has been executed at least once
	AtLeastLag(B_1, B_2, n)	AtLeastLag(AtLeast(Give painkiller, 1), AtLeast(Take anticoagulants, 1), 12): if Give painkiller is executed at least once, then at least 12 time units have to have passed before Take anticoagulants can be executed at least once
Resource	AtLeastAvailable(I, n)	AtLeastAvailable(nurse, 2): there should be at least 2 nurses available to the process (but they are allowed to be in use by the process).
	AtMostAvailable(I, n)	AtMostAvailable(nurse, 4): there should be no more than 4 nurses available to the process
	AtLeastUsage(act, I, n)	AtLeastUsage(Register patient, receptionist, 1): at least 1 receptionist is needed to execute Register patient
	AtMostUsage(act, I, n)	AtMostUsage(Register patient, receptionist, 2): no more than 2 receptionists should be used to execute Register patient
	(No) ActivityAuthorization (I, act)	ActivityAuthorization(doctor, Clinical exam): a doctor is allowed to execute a Clinical exam

References

Dumas, M., La Rosa, M., Mendling, J., Reijers, H.A.: Fundamentals of Business Process Management. Springer, Heidelberg (2018). https://doi.org/10.1007/978-3-662-56509-4

Trkman, P.: The critical success factors of business process management. Int. J. Inf. Manag. **30**, 125–134 (2010)

Weske, M.: Business Process Management: Concepts, Languages, Architectures. Springer, Heidelberg (2012). https://doi.org/10.1007/978-3-642-28616-2

Guha, S., Kettinger, W.J., Teng, J.T.C.: Business process reengineering. Inf. Syst. Manag. **10**, 13–22 (1993)

Strnadl, C.F.: Aligning business and IT: the process-driven architecture model. Inf. Syst. Manag. **23**, 67–77 (2006)

Di Ciccio, C., Marrella, A., Russo, A.: Knowledge-intensive processes: characteristics, requirements and analysis of contemporary approaches. J. Data Semant. **4**(1), 29–57 (2014). https://doi.org/10.1007/s13740-014-0038-4

van der Aalst, W.M.P.: Business process management: a comprehensive survey. ISRN Softw. Eng. **2013**, 1–37 (2013)

Reichert, M., Weber, B.: Enabling Flexibility in Process-Aware Information Systems: Challenges, Methods, Technologies. Springer, Heidelberg (2012). https://doi.org/10.1007/978-3-642-30409-5

Recker, J., Rosemann, M., Indulska, M., Green, P.: Business process modeling- a comparative analysis. J. Assoc. Inf. Syst. **10**, 333–363 (2009)

van der Aalst, W.M.P.: Process Mining: Discovery, Conformance and Enhancement of Business Processes. Springer, Heidelberg (2011). https://doi.org/10.1007/978-3-642-19345-3

van der Aalst, W.M.P., et al.: Process mining manifesto. In: Daniel, F., Barkaoui, K., Dustdar, S. (eds.) BPM 2011. LNBIP, vol. 99, pp. 169–194. Springer, Heidelberg (2012). https://doi.org/10.1007/978-3-642-28108-2_19

van der Aalst, W.M.P.: Process-aware information systems: lessons to be learned from process mining. In: Jensen, K., van der Aalst, W.M.P. (eds.) Transactions on Petri Nets and Other Models of Concurrency II. LNCS, vol. 5460, pp. 1–26. Springer, Heidelberg (2009). https://doi.org/10.1007/978-3-642-00899-3_1

Vassilakopoulou, P., Ponis, S.T., Gayialis, S.P., Papadopoulos, G.A., Tatsiopoulos, I.P.: Integrating process modeling and simulation with benchmarking using a business process management system for local government. Int. J. Comput. Theory Eng. **8**, 482–489 (2015)

Lenz, R., Reichert, M.: IT support for healthcare processes - premises, challenges, perspectives. Data Knowl. Eng. **61**, 39–58 (2007)

Vanhaecht, K., De Witte, K., Depreitere, R., Sermeus, W.: Clinical pathway audit tools: a systematic review. J. Nurs. Manag. **14**, 529–537 (2006)

Goedertier, S., Vanthienen, J., Caron, F.: Declarative business process modelling: Principles and modelling languages. Enterp. Inf. Syst. **9**, 161–185 (2015)

van der Aalst, W.M.P., Pesic, M., Schonenberg, H.: Declarative workflows: balancing between flexibility and support. Comput. Sci. - Res. Dev. **23**, 99–113 (2009)

Rovani, M., Maggi, F.M., de Leoni, M., van der Aalst, W.M.P.: Declarative process mining in healthcare. Expert Syst. Appl. **42**, 9236–9251 (2015)

Curtis, B., Kellner, M.I., Over, J.: Process modeling. Commun. ACM – Spec. Issue Anal. Model. Softw. Dev. **35**, 75–90 (1992)

Schonenberg, H., Mans, R., Russell, N., Mulyar, N., van der Aalst, W.M.P.: Process flexibility: a survey of contemporary approaches. In: Dietz, J.L.G., Albani, A., Barjis, J. (eds.) CIAO!/ EOMAS -2008. LNBIP, vol. 10, pp. 16–30. Springer, Heidelberg (2008). https://doi.org/10. 1007/978-3-540-68644-6_2

Borrego, D., Barba, I.: Conformance checking and diagnosis for declarative business process models in data-aware scenarios. Expert Syst. Appl. **41**, 5340–5352 (2014)

Pesic, M.: Constraint-based workflow management systems: shifting control to users (2008)

Mukkamala, R.R.: A formal model for declarative workflows - dynamic condition response graphs (2012)

Debois, S., Hildebrandt, T.T., Laursen, P.H., Ulrik, K.R.: Declarative process mining for DCR graphs, pp. 759–764 (2017)

Maggi, F.M.: Discovering metric temporal business constraints from event logs. In: Johansson, B., Andersson, B., Holmberg, N. (eds.) BIR 2014. LNBIP, vol. 194, pp. 261–275. Springer, Cham (2014). https://doi.org/10.1007/978-3-319-11370-8_19

Burattin, A., Maggi, F.M., van der Aalst, W.M.P., Sperduti, A.: Techniques for a posteriori analysis of declarative processes. In: 2012 IEEE EDOC, Beijing, China, pp. 41–50 (2012)

Maggi, F.M.: Declarative process mining with the declare component of ProM. In: CEUR, vol. 1021 (2013)

Maggi, F.M., Di Ciccio, C., Di Francescomarino, C., Kala, T.: Parallel algorithms for the automated discovery of declarative process models. Inf. Syst. **74**, 136–152 (2018)

Maggi, F.M., Bose, R.P.J.C., van der Aalst, W.M.P.: Efficient discovery of understandable declarative process models from event logs. In: Ralyté, J., Franch, X., Brinkkemper, S., Wrycza, S. (eds.) CAiSE 2012. LNCS, vol. 7328, pp. 270–285. Springer, Heidelberg (2012). https://doi.org/10.1007/978-3-642-31095-9_18

Di Ciccio, C., Schouten, M.H.M., de Leoni, M., Mendling, J.: Declarative process discovery with MINERful in ProM. In: CEUR, vol. 1418, pp. 60–64 (2015)

Di Ciccio, C., Maggi, F.M., Mendling, J.: Efficient discovery of target-branched declare constraints. Inf. Syst. **56**, 258–283 (2016)

De Smedt, J., De Weerdt, J., Vanthienen, J.: Fusion miner: process discovery for mixed-paradigm models. Decis. Support Syst. **77**, 123–136 (2015)

vanden Broucke, S.K.L.M., Vanthienen, J., Baesens, B.: Declarative process discovery with evolutionary computing. In: Proceedings of the 2014 IEEE Congress on Evolutionary Computation CEC 2014, pp. 2412–2419 (2014)

Rebuge, Á., Ferreira, D.R.: Business process analysis in healthcare environments: a methodology based on process mining. Inf. Syst. **37**, 99–116 (2012)

van Eck, M.L., Lu, X., Leemans, S.J.J., van der Aalst, W.M.P.: PM^2: a process mining project methodology. In: Zdravkovic, J., Kirikova, M., Johannesson, P. (eds.) CAiSE 2015. LNCS, vol. 9097, pp. 297–313. Springer, Cham (2015). https://doi.org/10.1007/978-3-319-19069-3_19

Haisjackl, C., Barba, I., Zugal, S., Soffer, P., Hadar, I., Reichert, M., Pinggera, J., Weber, B.: Understanding declare models: strategies, pitfalls, empirical results. Softw. Syst. Model. **15** (2), 1–28 (2014). https://doi.org/10.1007/s10270-014-0435-z

Hollingsworth, D.: The Workflow Reference Model (1995)

Hevner, A.R., March, S.T., Park, J., Ram, S.: Design science in information systems research. MIS Q. **28**, 75–105 (2004)

Peffers, K., Tuunanen, T., Rothenberger, M.A., Chatterjee, S.: A design science research methodology for information systems research. J. Manag. Inf. Syst. **24**, 45–77 (2007)

Wieringa, R.J.: Design science as nested problem solving. In: Proceedings of the 4th International Conference on Design Science Research in Information Systems and Technology - DESRIST 2009, pp. 1–12. ACM Press, New York (2009)

Wieringa, R.J., Heerkens, J.M.G.: The methodological soundness of requirements engineering papers: a conceptual framework and two case studies. Requir. Eng. **11**, 295–307 (2006)

Sein, M.K., Henfridsson, O., Purao, S., Rossi, M., Lindgren, R.: Action design research. MIS Q. **35**, 37–56 (2011)

Lu, R., Sadiq, S.W.: A survey of comparative business process modeling approaches. In: Abramowicz, W. (ed.) BIS 2007. LNCS, vol. 4439, pp. 82–94. Springer, Heidelberg (2007). https://doi.org/10.1007/978-3-540-72035-5_7

Krogstie, J.: Perspectives to process modeling. In: Glykas, M. (ed.) BPM. SCI, vol. 444, pp. 1–39. Springer, Heidelberg (2013). https://doi.org/10.1007/978-3-642-28409-0_1

White, S.A.: Introduction to BPMN, pp. 1–11. IBM Cooperation (2004)

Object Management Group: Unified Modeling Language (UML) (2015)

Rowley, J.: The wisdom hierarchy: representations of the DIKW hierarchy. J. Inf. Sci. **33**, 163–180 (2007)

Ferreira, H.M., Ferreira, D.R.: An integrated life cycle for workflow management based on learning and planning. Int. J. Coop. Inf. Syst. **15**, 485–505 (2006)

Object Management Group: Decision Model and Notation (DMN1.1) (2016)

Shostack, G.L.: Positioning through structural change. J. Mark. **51**, 34–43 (1987)

Wastell, D.G., White, P., Kawalek, P.: A methodology for business process redesign: experiences and issues. J. Strateg. Inf. Syst. **3**, 23–40 (1994)

Slaats, T., Mukkamala, R.R., Hildebrandt, T., Marquard, M.: Exformatics declarative case management workflows as DCR graphs. In: Daniel, F., Wang, J., Weber, B. (eds.) BPM 2013. LNCS, vol. 8094, pp. 339–354. Springer, Heidelberg (2013). https://doi.org/10.1007/978-3-642-40176-3_28

Hull, R., Damaggio, E., Fournier, F., Gupta, M., Heath, F., Hobson, S., Linehan, M.H., Maradugu, S., Nigam, A., Sukaviriya, P., Vaculin, R.: Introducing the guard-stage-milestone approach for specifying business entity lifecycles. In: Bravetti, M., Bultan, T. (eds.) WS-FM 2010. LNCS, vol. 6551, pp. 1–24. Springer, Heidelberg (2010). https://doi.org/10.1007/978-3-642-19589-1_1

Nelson, H.J., Poels, G., Genero, M., Piattini, M.: A conceptual modeling quality framework. Softw. Qual. J. **20**, 201–228 (2012)

Mertens, S., Gailly, F., Poels, G.: Enhancing declarative process models with DMN decision logic. In: Gaaloul, K., Schmidt, R., Nurcan, S., Guerreiro, S., Ma, Q. (eds.) CAISE 2015. LNBIP, vol. 214, pp. 151–165. Springer, Cham (2015). https://doi.org/10.1007/978-3-319-19237-6_10

Moody, D.L.: The "physics" of notations: toward a scientific basis for constructing visual notations in software engineering. IEEE Trans. Softw. Eng. **35**, 756–779 (2009)

Wand, Y., Storey, V.C., Weber, R.: An ontological analysis of the relationship construct in conceptual modeling. ACM Trans. Database Syst. **24**, 494–528 (1999)

Guizzardi, G.: Ontology-based evaluation and design of visual conceptual modeling languages. In: Reinhartz-Berger, I., Sturm, A., Clark, T., Cohen, S., Bettin, J. (eds.) Domain Engineering: Product Lines, Languages and Conceptual Models, pp. 317–347. Springer, Heidelberg (2013). https://doi.org/10.1007/978-3-642-36654-3_13

Fahland, D., Lübke, D., Mendling, J., Reijers, H., Weber, B., Weidlich, M., Zugal, S.: Declarative versus imperative process modeling languages: the issue of understandability. In: Halpin, T.A., Krogstie, J., Nurcan, S., Proper, E., Schmidt, R., Soffer, P., Ukor, R. (eds.) BPMDS/EMMSAD -2009. LNBIP, vol. 29, pp. 353–366. Springer, Heidelberg (2009). https://doi.org/10.1007/978-3-642-01862-6_29

Object Management Group: Business Process Model and Notation (BPMN2.02) (2013)

Petri, C.A.: Kommunikation mit automaten (1962)

Murata, T.: Petri nets: properties, analysis and applications. Proc. IEEE **77**, 541–580 (1989)

Mulyar, N., Pesic, M., van der Aalst, W.M.P., Peleg, M.: Declarative and procedural approaches for modelling clinical guidelines: addressing flexibility issues. In: ter Hofstede, A., Benatallah, B., Paik, H.-Y. (eds.) BPM 2007. LNCS, vol. 4928, pp. 335–346. Springer, Heidelberg (2008). https://doi.org/10.1007/978-3-540-78238-4_35

Lu, R., Sadiq, S.W., Governatori, G.: On managing business processes variants. Data Knowl. Eng. **68**, 642–664 (2009)

Bernardi, M.L., Cimitile, M., Di Lucca, G., Maggi, F.M.: Using declarative workflow languages to develop process-centric Web Applications. In: Proceedings of IEEE International EDOC 2012 Workshops, Beijing, China, pp. 56–65 (2012)

Montali, M.: Specification and Verification of Declarative Open Interaction Models. LNBIP, vol. 56. Springer, Heidelberg (2010). https://doi.org/10.1007/978-3-642-14538-4

Caron, F., Vanthienen, J., Baesens, B.: Comprehensive rule-based compliance checking and risk management with process mining. Decis. Support Syst. **54**, 1357–1369 (2013)

Dadam, P., Reichert, M., Kuhn, K.: Clinical workflows - the killer application for process-oriented information systems? In: Abramowicz, W., Orlowska, M.E. (eds.) BIS 2000, pp. 36–59. Springer, London (2000). https://doi.org/10.1007/978-1-4471-0761-3_3

Lanz, A., Weber, B., Reichert, M.: Time patterns for process-aware information systems. Requirements Eng. **19**(2), 113–141 (2012). https://doi.org/10.1007/s00766-012-0162-3

Barba, I., Lanz, A., Weber, B., Reichert, M., Del Valle, C.: Optimized time management for declarative workflows. In: Bider, I., et al. (eds.) BPMDS/EMMSAD -2012. LNBIP, vol. 113, pp. 195–210. Springer, Heidelberg (2012). https://doi.org/10.1007/978-3-642-31072-0_14

Westergaard, M., Maggi, F.M.: Looking into the future. In: Meersman, R., Panetto, H., Dillon, T., Rinderle-Ma, S., Dadam, P., Zhou, X., Pearson, S., Ferscha, A., Bergamaschi, S., Cruz, I. F. (eds.) OTM 2012. LNCS, vol. 7565, pp. 250–267. Springer, Heidelberg (2012). https://doi.org/10.1007/978-3-642-33606-5_16

Debois, S., Hildebrandt, T., Slaats, T.: Concurrency and asynchrony in declarative workflows. In: Motahari-Nezhad, H.R., Recker, J., Weidlich, M. (eds.) BPM 2015. LNCS, vol. 9253, pp. 72–89. Springer, Cham (2015). https://doi.org/10.1007/978-3-319-23063-4_5

Lenz, R., Peleg, M., Reichert, M.: Healthcare process support: achievements, challenges, current research. Int. J. Knowl.-Based Organ. **2**(4), 784–795 (2012)

Montali, M., Chesani, F., Mello, P., Maggi, F.M.: Towards data-aware constraints in declare. In: Proceedings of the 28th Annual ACM Symposium on Applied Computing. SAC, pp. 1391–1396. ACM Press, New York (2013)

Maggi, F.M., Dumas, M., García-Bañuelos, L., Montali, M.: Discovering data-aware declarative process models from event logs. In: Daniel, F., Wang, J., Weber, B. (eds.) BPM 2013. LNCS, vol. 8094, pp. 81–96. Springer, Heidelberg (2013). https://doi.org/10.1007/978-3-642-40176-3_8

Taylor, J., Fish, F.A., Vanthienen, J.: Emerging standards in decision modeling - an introduction to decision model & notation. In: iBPMS: Intelligent BPM Systems: Intelligent BPM Systems: Impact and Opportunity, pp. 133–146 (2013)

van der Aa, H., Leopold, H., Batoulis, K., Weske, M., Reijers, Hajo A.: Integrated process and decision modeling for data-driven processes. In: Reichert, M., Reijers, Hajo A. (eds.) BPM 2015. LNBIP, vol. 256, pp. 405–417. Springer, Cham (2016). https://doi.org/10.1007/978-3-319-42887-1_33

Codasyl: A modern appraisal of decision tables. In: Report of the Decision Table Task Group, pp. 230–232. ACM, New York (1982)

Vanthienen, J.: Introducing a proposal to standardize a Decision Model and Notation (2014)

Russell, N., ter Hofstede, A.H.M., Edmond, D., van der Aalst, W.M.P.: Workflow resource patterns (2004)

Russell, N., van der Aalst, W.M.P., ter Hofstede, A.H.M., Edmond, D.: Workflow resource patterns: identification, representation and tool support. In: Pastor, O., Falcão e Cunha, J. (eds.) CAiSE 2005. LNCS, vol. 3520, pp. 216–232. Springer, Heidelberg (2005). https://doi.org/10.1007/11431855_16

Mulyar, N.: Pattern-based evaluation of Oracle-BPEL (v.10.1.2). Technical report BPM-05-24, BPMcenter.org (2005)

Wohed, P., Russell, N., ter Hofstede, A.H.M., Andersson, B., van der Aalst, W.M.P.: Patterns-based evaluation of open source BPM systems: the cases of jBPM, OpenWFE, and Enhydra Shark. Inf. Softw. Technol. **51**, 1187–1216 (2009)

Jiménez-Ramírez, A., Barba, I., del Valle, C., Weber, B.: Generating multi-objective optimized business process enactment plans. In: Salinesi, C., Norrie, M.C., Pastor, Ó. (eds.) CAiSE 2013. LNCS, vol. 7908, pp. 99–115. Springer, Heidelberg (2013). https://doi.org/10.1007/978-3-642-38709-8_7

ISO/IEC: ISO/IEC 9075-2:2011(en): Information technology - Database languages - SQL - Part 2: Foundation (SQL/Foundation) (2011)

Peffers, K., Rothenberger, M.A., Tuunanen, T., Vaezi, R.: Design science research evaluation. In: Peffers, K., Rothenberger, M., Kuechler, B. (eds.) DESRIST 2012. LNCS, vol. 7286, pp. 398–410. Springer, Heidelberg (2012). https://doi.org/10.1007/978-3-642-29863-9_29

Krogstie, J.: Evaluating UML: a practical application of a framework for the understanding of quality in requirements specifications and conceptual modeling. In: Norwegian Informatics Conference (NIK) (2000)

Rotter, T., et al.: Clinical pathways: effects on professional practice, patient outcomes, length of stay and hospital costs. Cochrane Database Syst. Rev. **3**, 1–170 (2010)

Maggi, F.M., Mooij, A.J., van der Aalst, W.M.P.: User-guided discovery of declarative process models. In: IEEE Symposium on Computational Intelligence and Data Mining CIDM, pp. 192–199 (2011)

Jensen, K.: Coloured petri nets. In: Brauer, W., Reisig, W., Rozenberg, G. (eds.) ACPN 1986. LNCS, vol. 254, pp. 248–299. Springer, Heidelberg (1997). https://doi.org/10.1007/978-3-540-47919-2_10

Sadiq, S.W., Orlowska, M.E., Sadiq, W.: Specification and validation of process constraints for flexible workflows. Inf. Syst. **30**, 349–378 (2005)

De Smedt, J., De Weerdt, J., Vanthienen, J., Poels, G.: Mixed-paradigm process modeling with intertwined state spaces. Bus. Inf. Syst. Eng. **58**, 19–29 (2016)

Maggi, F.M., Slaats, T., Reijers, H.A.: The automated discovery of hybrid processes. In: Sadiq, S., Soffer, P., Völzer, H. (eds.) BPM 2014. LNCS, vol. 8659, pp. 392–399. Springer, Cham (2014a). https://doi.org/10.1007/978-3-319-10172-9_27

Frank, U.: Multi-perspective enterprise modeling: foundational concepts, prospects and future research challenges. Softw. Syst. Model. **13**, 941–962 (2014)

Madhavji, N.H., Schafer, W.: Prism - methodology and process-oriented environment. IEEE Trans. Softw. Eng. **17**, 1270–1283 (1991)

Di Ciccio, C., Maggi, F.M., Montali, M., Mendling, J.: Ensuring model consistency in declarative process discovery. In: Motahari-Nezhad, H.R., Recker, J., Weidlich, M. (eds.) BPM 2015. LNCS, vol. 9253, pp. 144–159. Springer, Cham (2015). https://doi.org/10.1007/978-3-319-23063-4_9

Di Ciccio, C., Mecella, M.: On the discovery of declarative control flows for artful processes. ACM Trans. Manag. Inf. Syst. **5**, 24, 1–24, 37 (2015)

Maggi, F.M., Bose, R.P.J.C., van der Aalst, W.M.P.: A knowledge-based integrated approach for discovering and repairing declare maps. In: Salinesi, C., Norrie, M.C., Pastor, Ó. (eds.) CAiSE 2013. LNCS, vol. 7908, pp. 433–448. Springer, Heidelberg (2013). https://doi.org/10.1007/978-3-642-38709-8_28

Netto, J.M., Barboza, T., Baião, F.A., Santoro, F.M.: KiPN: a visual notation for knowledge-intensive processes. Int. J. Bus. Process Integr. Manag. **9**, 197–219 (2019)

Payton, F.C., Paré, G., LeRouge, C., Reddy, M.: Health care IT: process, people, patients and interdisciplinary considerations. J. Assoc. Inf. Syst. **12**(2), 1–13 (2011)

Anyanwu, K., Sheth, A.P., Cardoso, J., Miller, J.A., Kochut, K.J.: Healthcare enterprise process development and integration. J. Res. Pract. Inf. Technol. **35**, 83–98 (2003)

Lillrank, P., Liukko, M.: Standard, routine and non-routine processes in health care. Int. J. Health Care Qual. Assur. **17**, 39–46 (2004)

Birkmeyer, J.D., Finlayson, E.V.A., Birkmeyer, C.M.: Volume standards for high-risk surgical procedures: potential benefits of the Leapfrog initiative. Surgery **130**, 415–422 (2001)

Gawande, A.: The Checklist Manifesto: How to Get Things Right. Metropolitan Books (2009)

De Bleser, L., Depreitere, R., De Waele, K., Vanhaecht, K., Vlayen, J., Sermeus, W.: Defining pathways. J. Nurs. Manag. **14**, 553–563 (2006)

Campbell, H., Hotchkiss, R., Bradshaw, N., Porteous, M.: Integrated care pathways. BMJ **316**, 133 (1998)

Keel, G., Savage, C., Rafiq, M., Mazzocato, P.: Time-driven activity-based costing in health care: a systematic review of the literature. Health Policy (New York) **121**, 755–763 (2017)

Amorim Lopes, M., Soares, C., Almeida, Á., Almada-Lobo, B.: Comparing comparables: an approach to accurate cross-country comparisons of health systems for effective healthcare planning and policy guidance. Health Syst. **5**, 192–212 (2016). https://doi.org/10.1057/hs.2015.21

Faber, B., Konrad, R.A., Tang, C., Trapp, A.C.: Examining the impact of regular physician visits on heart failure patients: a use case with electronic health data. Health Syst. **5**, 132–139 (2016)

Hofmann, P.B., Perry, F.: Management Mistakes in Healthcare: Identification, Correction, and Prevention. Cambridge University Press, Cambridge (2010)

Mazzocato, P., Savage, C., Brommels, M., Aronsson, H., Thor, J.: Lean thinking in healthcare: a realist review of the literature. BMJ Qual. Saf. **19**, 376–382 (2010)

Helfert, M.: Challenges of business processes management in healthcare: experience in the Irish healthcare sector. Bus. Process Manag. J. **15**, 937–952 (2009)

Rojo, M.G., et al.: Implementation of the Business Process Modelling Notation (BPMN) in the modelling of anatomic pathology processes. Diagn. Pathol. **3**(Suppl 1), S22 (2008)

Svagård, I., Farshchian, B.A.: Using business process modelling to model integrated care processes: experiences from a European project. In: Omatu, S., Rocha, M.P., Bravo, J., Fernández, F., Corchado, E., Bustillo, A., Corchado, J.M. (eds.) IWANN 2009. LNCS, vol. 5518, pp. 922–925. Springer, Heidelberg (2009). https://doi.org/10.1007/978-3-642-02481-8_140

Noumeir, R.: Radiology interpretation process modeling. J. Biomed. Inform. **39**, 103–114 (2006)

Braun, R., Schlieter, H., Burwitz, M., Esswein, W.: BPMN4CP: design and implementation of a BPMN extension for clinical pathways. In: IEEE BIBM 2014, pp. 9–16 (2014)

Aguilar, E.R., et al.: Process modeling of the health sector using BPMN: a case study. In: HEALTHINF 2008, pp. 173–178 (2008)

Putman, K., Anstey, A., Harper, P.R., Knight, V.A: Modelling of psoriasis patient flows for the reconfiguration of secondary care services and treatments. Heal. Syst. **5**(1), 13–20 (2016)

Mans, R.S., Schonenberg, M.H., Song, M., van der Aalst, W.M.P., Bakker, P.J.M.: Application of process mining in healthcare – a case study in a Dutch hospital. In: Fred, A., Filipe, J., Gamboa, H. (eds.) BIOSTEC 2009. CCIS, vol. 25, pp. 425–438. Springer, Heidelberg (2009). https://doi.org/10.1007/978-3-540-92219-3_32

Rismanchian, F., Lee, Y.H.: Process mining-based method of designing and optimizing the layouts of emergency departments in hospitals. Heal. Environ. Res. Des. J. **10**, 105–120 (2017)

Rashid, M., Naeem, H., Aamir, M., Ali, W., Ahmed, W.: A multi-level process mining framework for correlating and clustering of biomedical activities using event logs. Int. J. Adv. Comput. Sci. Appl. **8**, 393–401 (2017)

Rojas, E., Munoz-Gama, J., Sepúlveda, M., Capurro, D.: Process mining in healthcare: a literature review. J. Biomed. Inform. **61**, 224–236 (2016)

Huang, Z., Dong, W., Ji, L., Gan, C., Lu, X., Duan, H.: Discovery of clinical pathway patterns from event logs using probabilistic topic models. J. Biomed. Inform. **47**, 39–57 (2014)

Huang, Z., Dong, W., Bath, P., Ji, L., Duan, H.: On mining latent treatment patterns from electronic medical records. Data Min. Knowl. Discov. **29**(4), 914–949 (2014). https://doi.org/10.1007/s10618-014-0381-y

Wang, T., Tian, X., Yu, M., Qi, X., Yang, L.: Stage division and pattern discovery of complex patient care processes. J. Syst. Sci. Complex. **30**(5), 1136–1159 (2017). https://doi.org/10.1007/s11424-017-5302-x

Lismont, J., Janssens, A.S., Odnoletkova, I., vanden Broucke, S., Caron, F., Vanthienen, J.: A guide for the application of analytics on healthcare processes: a dynamic view on patient pathways. Comput. Biol. Med. **77**, 125–134 (2016)

Schönig, S., Di Ciccio, C., Maggi, F.M., Mendling, J.: Discovery of multi-perspective declarative process models. In: Sheng, Q.Z., Stroulia, E., Tata, S., Bhiri, S. (eds.) ICSOC 2016. LNCS, vol. 9936, pp. 87–103. Springer, Cham (2016). https://doi.org/10.1007/978-3-319-46295-0_6

Agrawal, R., Srikant, R.: Fast algorithms for mining association rules. In: VLDB, pp. 487–499 (1994)

Mitchell, M.: Introduction to Genetic Algorithms. MIT Press, Cambridge (1996)

Johnson, A.E.W., et al.: MIMIC-III, a freely accessible critical care database. Sci. Data. **3**, 160035 (2016)

Dijkman, R., Lammers, S.V., de Jong, A.: Properties that influence business process management maturity and its effect on organizational performance. Inf. Syst. Front. **18**(4), 717–734 (2015). https://doi.org/10.1007/s10796-015-9554-5

Hertz, S., Johansson, J.K., de Jager, F.: Customer-oriented cost cutting: process management at Volvo. Supply Chain Manag. **6**, 128–142 (2001)

Kim, G., Suh, Y.: Semantic business process space for intelligent management of sales order business processes. Inf. Syst. Front. **13**, 515–542 (2011)

Krishnan, M.S., Mukhopadhyay, T., Zubrow, D.: Software process models and project performance. Inf. Syst. Front. **1**, 267–277 (1999)

Palvia, P., Lowe, K., Nemati, H., Jacks, T.: Information technology issues in healthcare: hospital CEO and CIO perspectives. Inf. Technol. **30**, 293–312 (2012)

Klein, J.H., Young, T.: Health care: a case of hypercomplexity? Health Syst. **4**, 104–110 (2015)

Mertens, S., Gailly, F., Poels, G.: Towards a decision-aware declarative process modeling language for knowledge-intensive processes. Expert Syst. Appl. **87**, 316–334 (2017)

Mardini, M.T., Ras, Z.W.: Discovering primary medical procedures and their associations with other procedures in HCUP data. Inf. Syst. Front. 1–15 (2020). https://doi.org/10.1007/s10796-020-10058-9

Greenes, R.A., Bates, D.W., Kawamoto, K., Middleton, B., Osheroff, J., Shahar, Y.: Clinical decision support models and frameworks: seeking to address research issues underlying implementation successes and failures. J. Biomed. Inform. **78**, 134–143 (2018)

Kimble, C., de Vasconcelos, J.B., Rocha, Á.: Competence management in knowledge intensive organizations using consensual knowledge and ontologies. Inf. Syst. Front. **18**(6), 1119–1130 (2016). https://doi.org/10.1007/s10796-016-9627-0

Kamsu-Foguem, B., Tchuenté-Foguem, G., Foguem, C.: Using conceptual graphs for clinical guidelines representation and knowledge visualization. Inf. Syst. Front. **16**(4), 571–589 (2012). https://doi.org/10.1007/s10796-012-9360-2

Zhang, Y., Padman, R., Patel, N.: Paving the COWpath: learning and visualizing clinical pathways from electronic health record data. J. Biomed. Inform. **58**, 186–197 (2015)

Combi, C., Oliboni, B., Gabrieli, A.: Conceptual modeling of clinical pathways: making data and processes connected. In: 15th Conference on Artificial Intelligence in Medicine (AIME), Pavia, Italy, pp. 57–62 (2015)

Huang, Z., Bao, Y., Dong, W., Lu, X., Duan, H.: Online treatment compliance checking for clinical pathways. J. Med. Syst. **38**(10), 1–14 (2014). https://doi.org/10.1007/s10916-014-0123-0

Lawal, A.K., Rotter, T., Kinsman, L., Machotta, A., Ronellenfitsch, U., Scott, S.D., Goodridge, D., Plishka, C., Groot, G.: What is a clinical pathway? Refinement of an operational definition to identify clinical pathway studies for a Cochrane systematic review. BMC Med. **14**, 1–5 (2016)

Heß, M., Kaczmarek, M., Frank, U., Podleska, L.-E., Taeger, G.: Towards a pathway-based clinical cancer registration in hospital information systems. In: Riaño, D., Lenz, R., Miksch, S., Peleg, M., Reichert, M., ten Teije, A. (eds.) KR4HC 2015. LNCS (LNAI), vol. 9485, pp. 80–94. Springer, Cham (2015). https://doi.org/10.1007/978-3-319-26585-8_6

Hay, M., Weisner, T.S., Subramanian, S., Duan, N., Niedzinski, E.J., Kravitz, R.L.: Harnessing experience: exploring the gap between evidence-based medicine and clinical practice. J. Eval. Clin. Pract. **14**, 707–713 (2008)

Antunes, P., Pino, J.A., Tate, M., Barros, A.: Eliciting process knowledge through process stories. Inf. Syst. Front. **22**(5), 1179–1201 (2019). https://doi.org/10.1007/s10796-019-09922-0

Bygstad, B., Øvrelid, E., Lie, T., Bergquist, M.: Developing and organizing an analytics capability for patient flow in a general hospital. Inf. Syst. Front. **22**(2), 353–364 (2019). https://doi.org/10.1007/s10796-019-09920-2

Helm, E., Paster, F.: First steps towards process mining in distributed health information systems. Int. J. Electron. Telecommun. **61**, 137–142 (2015)

Baker, K., et al.: Process mining routinely collected electronic health records to define real-life clinical pathways during chemotherapy. Int. J. Med. Inform. **103**, 32–41 (2017)

Basole, R.C., et al.: Understanding variations in pediatric asthma care processes in the emergency department using visual analytics. J. Am. Med. Inform. Assoc. **22**, 318–323 (2015)

Orellana Garcia, A., Perez Ramirez, Y.E., Armenteros Larrea, O.U.: Process mining in healthcare: analysis and modeling of processes in the emergency area. IEEE Lat. Am. Trans. **13**, 1612–1618 (2015)

Huang, Z., Dong, W., Ji, L., He, C., Duan, H.: Incorporating comorbidities into latent treatment pattern mining for clinical pathways. J. Biomed. Inform. **59**, 227–239 (2016)

Funkner, A.A., Yakovlev, A.N., Kovalchuk, S.V.: Towards evolutionary discovery of typical clinical pathways in electronic health records. Procedia Comput. Sci. **119**, 234–244 (2017)

Duma, D., Aringhieri, R.: An ad hoc process mining approach to discover patient paths of an Emergency Department. Flex. Serv. Manuf. J. **32**(1), 6–34 (2018). https://doi.org/10.1007/s10696-018-9330-1

Andersen, S.N., Broberg, O.: A framework of knowledge creation processes in participatory simulation of hospital work systems. Ergonomics **60**, 487–503 (2017)

Kovalchuk, S., Funkner, A., Metsker, O., Yakovlev, A.: Simulation of patient flow in multiple healthcare units using process and data mining techniques for model identification. J. Biomed. Inform. **82**, 128–142 (2018)

Abo-Hamad, W.: Patient pathways discovery and analysis using process mining techniques: an emergency department case study. In: Cappanera, P., Li, J., Matta, A., Sahin, E., Vandaele, N. J., Visintin, F. (eds.) ICHCSE 2017. SPMS, vol. 210, pp. 209–219. Springer, Cham (2017). https://doi.org/10.1007/978-3-319-66146-9_19

Rojas, E., Cifuentes, A., Burattin, A., Munoz-Gama, J., Sepúlveda, M., Capurro, D.: Performance analysis of emergency room episodes through process mining. Int. J. Environ. Res. Public Health. **16**, 1274 (2019)

Ghasemi, M., Amyot, D.: Process mining in healthcare: a systematised literature review. Int. J. Electron. Healthc. 9, (2016)

Rojas, E., Arias, M., Sepúlveda, M.: Clinical Processes and Its Data, What Can We Do with Them? In: HEALTHINF '15. pp. 642–647. SCITEPRESS - Science and Technology Publications (2015)

Kurniati, A.P., Johnson, O., Hogg, D., Hall, G.: Process mining in oncology: A literature review. In: ICICM 2016. pp. 291–297. IEEE (2016)

Hildebrandt, T., Mukkamala, R.R., Slaats, T.: Declarative Modelling and Safe Distribution of Healthcare Workflows. In: Liu, Z., Wassyng, A. (eds.) FHIES 2011. LNCS, vol. 7151, pp. 39–56. Springer, Heidelberg (2012). https://doi.org/10.1007/978-3-642-32355-3_3

Cognini, R., Corradini, F., Gnesi, S., Polini, A., Re, B.: Business process flexibility - a systematic literature review with a software systems perspective. Inf. Syst. Front. **20**(2), 343–371 (2016). https://doi.org/10.1007/s10796-016-9678-2

Kluza, K., Nalepa, G.J.: Formal model of business processes integrated with business rules. Inf. Syst. Front. **21**(5), 1167–1185 (2019). https://doi.org/10.1007/s10796-018-9826-y

Santoro, F.M., Slaats, T., Hildebrandt, T.T., Baiao, F.A.: DCR-KiPN a hybrid modeling approach for knowledge-intensive processes. In: Laender, A.H.F., Pernici, B., Lim, E.-P., de Oliveira, J.P.M. (eds.) ER 2019. LNCS, vol. 11788, pp. 153–161. Springer, Cham (2019). https://doi.org/10.1007/978-3-030-33223-5_13

Burattin, A., Maggi, F.M., Sperduti, A.: Conformance checking based on multi-perspective declarative process models. Expert Syst. Appl. **65**, 194–211 (2016)

Burattin, A., Cimitile, M., Maggi, F.M., Sperduti, A.: Online discovery of declarative process models from event streams. IEEE Trans. Serv. Comput. **8**, 833–846 (2015)

Shearer, C.: The CRISP-DM model: the new blueprint for data mining. J. Data Warehouse. **5**, 13–22 (2000)

Mariscal, G., Marbán, Ó., Fernández, C.: A survey of data mining and knowledge discovery process models and methodologies. Knowl. Eng. Rev. **25**, 137–166 (2010)

Manning, C.D., Schütze, H.: Foundations of Statistical Natural Language Processing. MIT Press, Cambridge (1999)

Daelemans, W., Zavrel, J., van Der Sloot, K., van Den Bosch, A.: TiMBL: Tilburg memory based learner, version 6.2, Reference Guide. Ilk Research Group, Technical report Ser. 66 (2009)

Di Ciccio, C., Mecella, M., Mendling, J.: The effect of noise on mined declarative constraints. In: Ceravolo, P., Accorsi, R., Cudre-Mauroux, P. (eds.) SIMPDA 2013. LNBIP, vol. 203, pp. 1–24. Springer, Heidelberg (2015). https://doi.org/10.1007/978-3-662-46436-6_1

Di Ciccio, C., Maggi, F.M., Montali, M., Mendling, J.: Resolving inconsistencies and redundancies in declarative process models. Inf. Syst. **64**, 425–446 (2017)

Guizzardi, G., Wagner, G., de Almeida Falbo, R., Guizzardi, R.S.S., Almeida, J.P.A.: Towards ontological foundations for the conceptual modeling of events. In: Ng, W., Storey, V.C., Trujillo, J.C. (eds.) ER 2013. LNCS, vol. 8217, pp. 327–341. Springer, Heidelberg (2013). https://doi.org/10.1007/978-3-642-41924-9_27

Braga, B.F.B., Almeida, J.P.A., Guizzardi, G., Benevides, A.B.: Transforming OntoUML into alloy: towards conceptual model validation using a lightweight formal method. Innov. Syst. Softw. Eng. **6**, 55–63 (2010)

Suriadi, S., Andrews, R., ter Hofstede, A.H.M., Wynn, M.T.: Event log imperfection patterns for process mining: towards a systematic approach to cleaning event logs. Inf. Syst. **64**, 132–150 (2017)

Rehse, J.-R., Fettke, P., Loos, P.: Process mining and the black swan: an empirical analysis of the influence of unobserved behavior on the quality of mined process models. In: Teniente, E., Weidlich, M. (eds.) BPM 2017. LNBIP, vol. 308, pp. 256–268. Springer, Cham (2018). https://doi.org/10.1007/978-3-319-74030-0_19

Deokar, A.V., El-Gayar, O.F.: Decision-enabled dynamic process management for networked enterprises. Inf. Syst. Front. **13**, 655–668 (2011)

Sittig, D.F., Wright, A., Osheroff, J.A., Middleton, B., Teich, J.M., Ash, J.S., Campbell, E., Bates, D.W.: Grand challenges in clinical decision support. J. Biomed. Inform. **41**, 387–392 (2008)

Nunes, V.T., Santoro, F.M., Werner, C.M.L., Ralha, C.G.: Context and planning for dynamic adaptation in PAIS. In: Reichert, M., Reijers, H.A. (eds.) BPM 2015. LNBIP, vol. 256, pp. 471–483. Springer, Cham (2016). https://doi.org/10.1007/978-3-319-42887-1_38

Fernandez-Llatas, C., Martinez-Millana, A., Martinez-Romero, A., Benedi, J.M., Traver, V.: Diabetes care related process modelling using process mining techniques. lessons learned in the application of interactive pattern recognition: coping with the spaghetti effect. In: 37th Annual International Conference of the IEEE Engineering in Medicine and Biology Society (EMBC), pp. 2127–2130. IEEE Xplore (2015)

Vanbrabant, L., Martin, N., Ramaekers, K., Braekers, K.: Quality of input data in emergency department simulations: framework and assessment techniques. Simul. Model. Pract. Theory **91**, 83–101 (2019)

van der Spoel, S., van Keulen, M., Amrit, C.: Process prediction in noisy data sets: a case study in a Dutch hospital. In: Cudre-Mauroux, P., Ceravolo, P., Gašević, D. (eds.) SIMPDA 2012. LNBIP, vol. 162, pp. 60–83. Springer, Heidelberg (2013). https://doi.org/10.1007/978-3-642-40919-6_4

Durieux, P., Nizard, R., Ravaud, P., Mounier, N., Lepage, E.: A clinical decision support system for prevention of venous thromboembolism. JAMA **283**, 2816–2821 (2000)

Martin, N., et al.: Recommendations for enhancing the usability and understandability of process mining in healthcare. Artif. Intell. Med. **109**, 101962 (2020)

Dumas, M., van der Aalst, W.M.P., ter Hofstede, A.H.M.: Process-Aware Information Systems: Bridging People and Software through Process Technology. Wiley, New York (2005)

Leymann, F., Roller, D.: Production Workflow - Concepts and Techniques. Prentice Hall PTR, Upper Saddle River (2000)

Pryss, R., Mundbrod, N., Langer, D., Reichert, M.: Supporting medical ward rounds through mobile task and process management. Inf. Syst. e-Bus. Manag. 107–146 (2015). https://doi.org/10.1007/s10257-014-0244-5

Lanz, A., Posenato, R., Combi, C., Reichert, M.: Controlling time-awareness in modularized processes. In: Schmidt, R., Guédria, W., Bider, I., Guerreiro, S. (eds.) BPMDS/EMMSAD - 2016. LNBIP, vol. 175, pp. 157–172. Springer, Cham (2014). https://doi.org/10.1007/978-3-319-39429-9_11

Haarmann, S., Podlesny, N.J., Hewelt, M., Meyer, A., Weske, M.: Production case management: a prototypical process engine to execute flexible business processes. In: Proceedings of the BPM Demo Session, pp. 110–114 (2015) van der Aalst, W.M.P.: Three good reasons for using a petri-net-based workflow management system. In: Wakayama, T., Kannapan, S., Khoong, C.M., Navathe, S., Yates, J. (eds.) Information and Process Integration in Enterprises. SECS, vol. 428, pp. 161–182. Springer, Boston (1998). https://doi.org/10.1007/978-1-4615-5499-8_10

Maggi, F.M., Montali, M., Di Ciccio, C., Mendling, J.: Semantical vacuity detection in declarative process mining. In: La Rosa, M., Loos, P., Pastor, O. (eds.) BPM 2016. LNCS, vol. 9850, pp. 158–175. Springer, Cham (2016). https://doi.org/10.1007/978-3-319-45348-4_10

Object Management Group: Decision Model and Notation (DMN1.0) (2014)

Ackermann, L., Schönig, S., Petter, S., Schützenmeier, N., Jablonski, S.: Execution of multi-perspective declarative process models. In: Panetto, H., Debruyne, C., Proper, H.A., Ardagna, C.A., Roman, D., Meersman, R. (eds.) OTM 2018. LNCS, vol. 11230, pp. 154–172. Springer, Cham (2018). https://doi.org/10.1007/978-3-030-02671-4_9

De Carvalho, R.M., Silva, N.C., Lima, R.M.F., Cornélio, M.L.: ReFlex: an efficient graph-based rule engine to execute declarative processes. In: 2013 IEEE International Conference on Systems, Man, and Cybernetics (SMC), pp. 1379–1384 (2013)

Marquard, M., Shahzad, M., Slaats, T.: Web-based modelling and collaborative simulation of declarative processes. In: Motahari-Nezhad, H., Recker, J., Weidlich, M. (eds.) BPM 2015. LNCS, vol. 9253, pp. 209–225. Springer, Cham (2015). https://doi.org/10.1007/978-3-319-23063-4_15

Benevides, A.B., Guizzardi, G., Braga, B.F.B., Almeida, J.P.A.: Validating modal aspects of OntoUML conceptual models using automatically generated visual word structures. J. Univers. Comput. Sci. **16**, 2904–2933 (2010)

Meier, J., Dietz, A., Boehm, A., Neumuth, T.: Predicting treatment process steps from events. J. Biomed. Inform. **53**, 308–319 (2015)

Mundbrod, N., Reichert, M.: Configurable and executable task structures supporting knowledge-intensive processes. In: Mayr, H.C., Guizzardi, G., Ma, H., Pastor, O. (eds.) ER 2017. LNCS, vol. 10650, pp. 388–402. Springer, Cham (2017). https://doi.org/10.1007/978-3-319-69904-2_30

Schonenberg, H., Weber, B., van Dongen, B., van der Aalst, W.: Supporting flexible processes through recommendations based on history. In: Dumas, M., Reichert, M., Shan, M.-C. (eds.) BPM 2008. LNCS, vol. 5240, pp. 51–66. Springer, Heidelberg (2008). https://doi.org/10.1007/978-3-540-85758-7_7

Barba, I., Weber, B., Del Valle, C., Jiménez-Ramírez, A.: User recommendations for the optimized execution of business processes. Data Knowl. Eng. **86**, 61–84 (2013)

Maggi, F.M., Di Francescomarino, C., Dumas, M., Ghidini, C.: Predictive monitoring of business processes. In: Jarke, M., Mylopoulos, J., Quix, C., Rolland, C., Manolopoulos, Y., Mouratidis, H., Horkoff, J. (eds.) CAiSE 2014. LNCS, vol. 8484, pp. 457–472. Springer, Cham (2014). https://doi.org/10.1007/978-3-319-07881-6_31

Metzger, A., et al.: Comparing and combining predictive business process monitoring techniques. IEEE Trans. Syst. Man Cybern. Syst. **45**, 276–290 (2015)

Di Francescomarino, C., Dumas, M., Maggi, F.M., Teinemaa, I.: Clustering-based predictive process monitoring. IEEE Trans. Serv. Comput. **12**(6), 896–909 (2019)

Evermann, J., Rehse, J.-R., Fettke, P.: A deep learning approach for predicting process behaviour at runtime. In: Dumas, M., Fantinato, M. (eds.) BPM 2016. LNBIP, vol. 281, pp. 327–338. Springer, Cham (2016). https://doi.org/10.1007/978-3-319-58457-7_24

Tax, N., Verenich, I., La Rosa, M., Dumas, M.: Predictive business process monitoring with LSTM neural networks. In: Dubois, E., Pohl, K. (eds.) CAiSE 2017. LNCS, vol. 10253, pp. 477–492. Springer, Cham (2017). https://doi.org/10.1007/978-3-319-59536-8_30

Song, M., Yang, H., Siadat, S.H., Pechenizkiy, M.: A comparative study of dimensionality reduction techniques to enhance trace clustering performances. Expert Syst. Appl. **40**, 3722–3737 (2013)

De Leoni, M., van der Aalst, W.M.P., Dees, M.: A general process mining framework for correlating, predicting and clustering dynamic behavior based on event logs. Inf. Syst. **56**, 235–257 (2016)

Song, M., Günther, C.W., van der Aalst, W.M.P.: Trace clustering in process mining. In: Ardagna, D., Mecella, M., Yang, J. (eds.) BPM 2008. LNBIP, vol. 17, pp. 109–120. Springer, Heidelberg (2009). https://doi.org/10.1007/978-3-642-00328-8_11

Tax, N., Teinemaa, I., van Zelst, S.J.: An interdisciplinary comparison of sequence modeling methods for next-element prediction. Softw. Syst. Model. **19**(6), 1345–1365 (2020). https://doi.org/10.1007/s10270-020-00789-3

Bajusz, D., Rácz, A., Héberger, K.: Why is Tanimoto index an appropriate choice for fingerprint-based similarity calculations? J. Cheminform. **7**(1), 1–13 (2015). https://doi.org/10.1186/s13321-015-0069-3

Ferri, C., Hernández-Orallo, J., Modroiu, R.: An experimental comparison of performance measures for classification. Pattern Recogn. Lett. **30**, 27–38 (2009)